THE

Essential Guide to

AROMATHERAPY

················· *and* ·················

VIBRATIONAL
HEALING

·······························

About the Author

Margaret Ann Lembo (Boynton Beach, FL) is a spiritual practitioner and owner of The Crystal Garden, a spiritual center and gift shop. For more than twenty-five years, she has led workshops and classes around the country. Her audio CDs (guided meditations and more) are distributed nationally. Visit her online at www.margaretannlembo.com.

To Write to the Author

If you wish to contact the author or would like more information about this book, please write to the author in care of Llewellyn Worldwide, and we will forward your request. Both the author and publisher appreciate hearing from you and learning of your enjoyment of this book and how it has helped you. Llewellyn Worldwide cannot guarantee that every letter written to the author can be answered, but all will be forwarded. Please write to:

Margaret Ann Lembo
℅ Llewellyn Worldwide
2143 Wooddale Drive
Woodbury, MN 55125-2989

Please enclose a self-addressed stamped envelope for reply,
or $1.00 to cover costs. If outside the USA, enclose
an international postal reply coupon.

Many of Llewellyn's authors have websites with additional
information and resources. For more information,
please visit our website at http://www.llewellyn.com.

THE

Essential Guide to

AROMATHERAPY

········· *and* ·········

VIBRATIONAL
HEALING

····························

AUTHOR OF
CHAKRA AWAKENING

MARGARET ANN LEMBO

Llewellyn Worldwide
Woodbury, Minnesota

First Edition
First Printing, 2016

Book design by Bob Gaul
Cover art by iStockphoto.com/15126330/©pawel.gaul
         iStockphoto.com/3491048/©claudelle
Cover design by Ellen Lawson
Editing by Patti Frazee
Interior scroll art by iStock.com/3491048/©claudelle

Llewellyn is a registered trademark of Llewellyn Worldwide Ltd.

Library of Congress Cataloging-in-Publication Data
Names: Lembo, Margaret Ann, 1957–
Title: The essential guide to aromatherapy and vibrational healing /
    Margaret Ann Lembo.
Description: First edition. | Woodbury, Minnesota : Llewellyn
Publications, 2016. | Includes guide to essential oils. | Includes bibliographical
    references and index.
Identifiers: LCCN 2015047702 (print) | LCCN 2015048960 (ebook) | ISBN
    9780738743394 | ISBN 9780738747781 ()
Subjects: LCSH: Vibration—Therapeutic use. | Aromatherapy. | Essences and
    essential oils.
Classification: LCC RM721 .L5135 2016 (print) | LCC RM721 (ebook) | DDC
    615.3/219—dc23
LC record available at http://lccn.loc.gov/2015047702

Llewellyn Worldwide Ltd. does not participate in, endorse, or have any authority or responsibility concerning private business transactions between our authors and the public.

All mail addressed to the author is forwarded, but the publisher cannot, unless specifically instructed by the author, give out an address or phone number.

Any Internet references contained in this work are current at publication time, but the publisher cannot guarantee that a specific location will continue to be maintained. Please refer to the publisher's website for links to authors' websites and other sources.

Llewellyn Publications
A Division of Llewellyn Worldwide Ltd.
2143 Wooddale Drive
Woodbury, MN 55125-2989
www.llewellyn.com

Printed in the United States of America

To my mother, Antoinette Lembo.
Thank you for teaching me to be one with the flowers
and garden. Thank you for teaching me to communicate
telepathically with nature. Thank you for being my mother!.

Contents

Part Two: The A-to-Z Essential Guide

*Essential Oil (Name); Key phrase; Botanical name; Note;
Method of extraction; Parts used; Fragrance; Color(s);
Chakra(s); Astrological sign(s); Planet(s); Number(s);
Animal(s); Element(s); Affirmation; Complementary flower
essences; Complementary stones; About the plant; Chemical
components; Spiritual uses; Mental uses; Emotional uses;
Physical uses; Therapeutic properties; Divine guidance;
For your safety; Interesting tidbits*

·····························

Part Three: Appendices

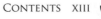

List of Essential Oils

Acknowledgments

This book has been a labor of love. I didn't want the process to end. Many wise people contributed to this book over the years while it was incubating in my consciousness.

My first thank-you goes out and up to my mother. Her love of gardening and reverence for the old ways provided me with the foundation for understanding and working with plants and creating aromatherapy recipes. Recipes, or formulas, are an integral piece of understanding and playing with oils. Fully experiencing their benefits also takes a solid connection to the plants, trees, and bushes on this glorious planet.

Thank you to everyone at Llewellyn Worldwide and especially Bill Krause, who had the vision and faith to publish my first book and continue to want more of my work. Thanks to all the editors at Llewellyn who have helped me grow as a writer and author. I have gratitude to Angela Wix, Elysia Gallo, and Carrie Obry.

An extra special thank-you is in order for my aromatherapy teacher and mentor, Dr. Annie Farrell. As a naturapath, Annie provided me with a deeper understanding of the oils and how to relate to them on a level I had not experienced until I was under her tutelage. It is because of her inspiration that I started my own private label line of oils at my store, The Crystal Garden. When I'm stuck or need ideas on how to tweak a scent for a certain purpose, Annie is the person I turn to for advice. She also taught me the real difference between the qualities of essential oils.

Geraldine Whidden was my first aromatherapy teacher. I was introduced to her line of oils in the early 1980s when I was still a banker. I am grateful for those early teachings. Thanks to Shellie Enteen, who provided me with an introduction to Bach Flower Remedies in the early 1990s. Thanks to Joan Ranquet, who is my true friend and fellow author. There is much comfort in having a good author friend while I write my books. I am grateful to have that comradery and support in my life!

A super special thank-you goes to Carol Killman Rosenberg, who is my personal editor. She knows how to polish my manuscripts, keep my voice, and make me look good to the publishers. Thank you, Kim Weiss, for introducing me to Carol. She is a gem, and I treasure her.

Thank you to everyone on the team at The Crystal Garden. Their good work, reliability, and dedication makes it possible for me to work from my home office while writing my books and creating affirmation decks and audio products. I can rest easy knowing that all is well. Special thanks to Pam Moore, Caitlin Ten Eyck, Dawn Seiler, Chrissy Clark, and Judy Waters, as well as Carmen Leidel, Marcie Hayunga, and Angelina Kessler. This amazing team also supports me as an author in social media and my book tours, along with Deanna Estes and Brandon Ellis in graphic design and web development.

Thank you to friends and family who believe in me and my work. Thanks to Mary Ann Garofala, Melissa Applegate, and Vickie Mitchell.

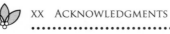

And most of all, thank you to my husband, Vincent. He is an inspiration and holds the space for me to do this work. Thank you, honey, for traveling this planet with me on book tours and selling my books and aromatherapy line at trade shows and expos. I really appreciate that you carry boxes and baggage, put up displays, and drive me around this planet to my appearances. Thank you for encouraging me to write the next book before I've even finished the one I am currently working on. I am blessed and grateful that you are the love of my life.

Thank you to all of the aromatherapists who wrote the books I've used as reference for many years. My sincere gratitude goes to Susan Worwood, Valerie Worwood, Wanda Sellar, Jennifer Peace Rhind, Julia Lawless, and Patricia Davis. Thanks for the dedication and knowledge of Robert Tisserand. His book *Essential Oil Safety, Second Edition* was an important reference along with his posts online as I researched the material for this book. These authors don't know me, but I feel like I know them. Thank you for your good work.

Introduction

This book is about using the aromatic parts of plants in the form of oils, mists, incense, and sprays for the purposes of healing physical, mental, and/ or emotional complaints and improving overall well-being. The uses described within this book are based on metaphysical principles (that which transcends the physical), as well as the physiological benefits provided by the chemical constituents within each essential oil. There are sixty essential oils described within these pages. Each essential oil and complementary vibrational tool discussed offers options for helping you to achieve spiritual, mental, and emotional balance. Singularly or in combination, they can be used as allies to assist you in staying focused on your intentions to escalate your self-awareness, achieve a state of balance and well-being, and create and maintain positive change in your life.

Establishing intention and accessing the unlimited potential provided by your imagination are important components of working with these vibrational teams. In this book, you will learn to develop a personal relationship with these tools. There are many layers to understanding vibrational healing. When it comes to aromatherapy and the energetic essence of the essential oils, it all starts with understanding how powerfully our sense of smell shapes our moods and behaviors. Aromas have an effect on our moods, decisions, and even on our ability to comprehend, remember, and process feelings and emotions. The limbic system of the brain is responsible for interpreting signals and influencing mood and emotion as well as serving as a storage area.

When an odor conjures up emotions, it also brings up memories. In fact, the sense of smell is the most powerful trigger of childhood memories. For instance, have you ever opened a box stored in the attic—maybe containing an old toy, Christmas decorations, or a holiday tablecloth—and the scent of whatever it is wafts from the box, flooding your consciousness with memories of a specific day or experience? The olfactory sense (our ability to process a smell) is the primary trigger of that memory. When I smell certain floral scents, I am immediately transported to my childhood garden. I am always grateful for the reminder, as my first and happiest memories are of time spent with my mother in that wonderful place.

We had a small front yard and backyard at our Brooklyn row house. In our neighborhood, trees lined the streets, and the backyards of the houses that backed up to our yard became a series of blooming gardens. Our garden was filled with many treasures—from pussy willows and forsythia to eggplants and tomatoes, and from azaleas and crocus to iris, lily of the valley, and sweet pea. My mother and I talked to the plants, weeded the garden, and nourished the soil with coffee grounds and eggshells.

The garden experience traveled with us to our summer home at the beach in Breezy Point, New York. It didn't occur to me until I was an adult that my mom—with me as her personal garden fairy—had actually grown an amazing garden in beach sand! Every year on Memorial Day weekend, we would leave Brooklyn to open the summer house and start the garden. On the way, we would pick up peat moss, cow manure, and starter plants. Once there, we would prepare the ground for the coming season. We would bury fish heads, kitchen cuttings from vegetables, and seaweed

I had collected from the shoreline to nourish and nurture the plants. Little did I know, we were composting. It was just what we did, and I am so grateful that these gardening experiences taught me to connect with the energy of the plants at a young age and to understand its value today.

I was happy to have the tasks of weeding and watering. With my hose in hand, I would imagine the plants with fully mature flowers or vegetables. I would make believe I was pouring nutrients and good energy into the roots through the water from the hose. I'd imagine I was part of the book *The Secret Garden*, working with my imaginary friends to bring the garden to life. *The Secret Garden* takes the reader on a journey in which faith restores health and flowers renew the spirit. This book and the many years of growing up in the garden inspired me to follow my spiritual path as well as to create my store and spiritual center, The Crystal Garden.

I believe in the magic of the garden and nature—plants, animals, fairies, and the elemental energies—as gifts from the earth to remember our soul contract and to recover our body, mind, and spirit.

The use of aromatherapy is a huge part of this litany of gifts from the earth. The extraction of the essential oil from the flower, plant, bark, and roots is just another level of receiving the magic of the garden and nature. I have used essential oils since the early 1980s to help me live a happier life. I used these fragrant essences when I was healing from the grief of my mother's passing. It was a huge relief to have hyacinth essential oil, along with many others, such as lavender, lemon, and bergamot, to restore my joy and to be able to look forward to life, even without my mother in it. It was a big rite of passage for me, and I am grateful for the opportunity to recover and rediscover myself with essential oils.

Essential oils have a true effect on activating memory and healing for inner peace and restoration. You can use an essential oil on many levels—for example, to relieve physical ailments such as respiratory challenges, to enhance your mental acuity, to heal emotional issues such as sadness or embarrassment, and/or to deepen a spiritual practice. Employ these scents as treasures provided to you by Mother Earth to support you on your journey here.

One of the goals of this book is to provide you with the know-how to change unconscious influences into conscious intentions. Accessing your memory bank and stored belief systems through the use of aromatherapy and its allies is an important tool for becoming self-aware. It can help you uncover pent-up emotions and feelings stored in your body, mind, or spirit at a time in your life when you are feeling blocked or heavy but don't know why. Recalling the memory of an emotional incident from childhood can be triggered by the scent of birch, vanilla, or cinnamon, for example. One scent may flood your consciousness with feelings of warmth and comfort, while another might call up anxiety and fear. The key is to remember the source or exact incident or series of events involved in that trigger in order to release it, heal it, and move on, free of the cords that had been binding you.

Over the years, I've taught many classes on aromatherapy. A favorite part of the class is the time spent concocting formulas based on the goals and intentions of the participants. This book will provide you the information you need to start your journey in learning to create your own formulas.

Through the sixty essential oils listed in the A-to-Z section of the book, you will learn which essential oils and complementary tools can assist you to heal, transform, and evolve on all levels—spiritually, mentally, emotionally, and physically. But first, in the following section, let's take a look at the prevalent role scents play in our spiritual journeys. Thereafter, you'll learn more about how to work with the essential oils and the other tools that can support you on your path.

Aromatherapy Safety

There are many opinions and diverse viewpoints on the safe use of essential oils. Through my research I have found that the most controversial subjects are the use of certain essential oils during pregnancy, the use of essential oils internally, and the use of essential oils with children. Professional organizations such as the National Association of Holistic Aromatherapy (NAHA) and the International Federation of Professional Aromatherapists (IFPA) post safety considerations and guidelines for the use of essential oils in all circumstances.

Inhalation, as a method of application, is a low-risk avenue for most people. Any risk associated with the inhalation method is from prolonged and excessive exposure to the oil vapors.

The age of an individual plays a part in determining the safe usage of essential oils. For example, infants and young children have a higher sensitivity to essential oils than adults. Safe dilutions, according to the NAHA, include "0.5–2.5% depending on the condition." It is best to avoid the use of birch, wintergreen, and peppermint with youngsters. Also, skin sensitivity is higher in the elderly population, so the dilution for topical application would be increased in such cases.

For the purposes of the use of aromatherapy as presented within this book, my recommendations are as follows:

- Avoid use of essential oils during pregnancy, especially during the first trimester. It has been shown that toxicity during pregnancy arises when certain essential oils are used in large doses. The key is to properly use essential oils as instructed by a skilled therapist. The cautious use of essential oils by a trained therapist can provide comfort and nurturance for a pregnant woman. According to Tisserand and Balacs, the following essential oils should not be used during pregnancy: wormwood, rue, oak moss, *Lavandula stoechas*, camphor, parsley seed, sage, and hyssop.

- Keep all essential oils out of the reach of children.

- Do not use essential oils on cats and dogs with short nasal canals like pugs, Boston Terriers, and many bulldogs. According to Joan Ranquet in *Energy Healing for Animals*, there is no distance between the nasal canal and brain and the delivery is extremely fast. More selective usage is possible by placing a little oil on a washcloth near their bed or food bowl.

- Do not use essential oils on birds.

- Keep essential oils away from the eyes.

- Do not use the same essential oil for prolonged periods.

- Avoid the use of undiluted essential oils on the skin.

- Avoid using essential oils internally.

- Some essential oils deteriorate plastic or other synthetic materials. Avoid contact with plastic or other synthetics.

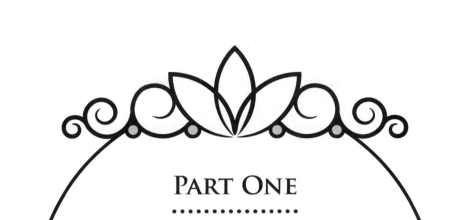

PART ONE

· · · · · · · · · · · · · · · ·

Understanding
the Basics of Your
Aromatherapy and
Vibrational Healing
Practices

CHAPTER ONE

• •

Working with Essential Oils

Essential oils have potent attributes on physical, mental, emotional, and spiritual levels. Through personal experience with aromatherapy, I have found relief from mental, emotional, and spiritual challenges, and I have witnessed the same in my clients. In this section, I will briefly introduce how the use of essential oils and aromatherapy evolved, and then I will move on to some helpful information for putting essential oils to work for you in your life for whatever changes you desire.

Historical Use of Essential Oils

Aromatic plants have played an important role in health, beauty, food preservation, and healing on all levels for millennia, with written records going back to around 3500 BC. Ancient Egyptians used aromatherapy in the embalming and mummification process (2650–2575 BC) as well as in their daily lives.

Still known today as master perfumers, the Egyptians were actually the first to extract the volatile oils from plants with the use of heat.

The earliest known Greek physician, Asclepius, who practiced around 1200 BC, combined the use of herbs with surgical procedures. According to Patricia Davis in her book *Aromatherapy: An A–Z*, the Greeks continued to perfect the process of extraction, eventually discovering a way to distill the volatile essences for use in their spiritual practices as well as for health and well-being. Persian philosopher Avicenna (c. 980–1035), known as the father of modern medicine and a pioneer in aromatherapy, is said to have further perfected the extraction process with the use of cooling systems in the distillation process.

The antiseptic, antibacterial, and antiviral properties of essential oils have been used to ward off diseases for centuries. It is said that during the Great Plague in Europe essential oils were used to prevent the plague from spreading. There were a number of these plagues that went through Seville (1647), London (1665–66), Vienna (1679), and Marseille (1720). Historical accounts suggest that because the perfumers were constantly handling aromatic substances in the making of perfumes, they were immune to this terrible illness.

René-Maurice Gattefossé (1881–1950), a French cosmetic chemist, is well known for his discovery of the use of lavender for burns. Gattefossé burned his hand while working in his laboratory and plunged his hand into the nearest tub of liquid, which was lavender oil. He noticed how quickly his burn healed, with minimal scarring. Because of this experience, he dedicated his life to uncovering the therapeutic qualities of the chemical components of essential oils. It was Gattefossé and his work that coined the term "aromatherapy" around 1928.

Another French practitioner, Jean Valnet (1920–1995), was inspired by the work of Gattefossé. Valnet used essential oils as a medical doctor during World War II in the treatment of battle wounds. His book *The Practice of Aromatherapy* evolved from his hands-on experiences and has become a true classic for all aromatherapists.

The Physical and Energetic Value of Essential Oils

These historical practitioners knew what we know today: Essential oils contain powerful chemical components. There is a considerable amount of scientific research supporting the ability of essential oils to deter a wide range of bacterial, fungal, viral, and/or other disease-causing microorganisms through the diffusion of oils into the atmosphere and onto the skin with the use of a carrier oil. When diffused, the scent particles of the oils also help to remove odors from the air as well as purify the surrounding atmosphere, in the case of environmental contaminants.

Essential oils also work on an energetic level to rebalance us spiritually, mentally, and emotionally, and offer many physiological benefits. Emotional and mental rebalancing includes raising our spirits when we are feeling down to clearing out negative thoughtforms as well as psychic debris. It is important to note here that thoughts create, or form, our reality; hence the term "thoughtforms." Throughout this book, I use this term to magnify for you the power of thoughts and intentions, as they create the world around us. "Psychic debris," another term you will encounter, is closely related and can be described as the energetic residue of unwanted negative thoughts, experiences, emotions, and feelings.

The energetic value, or vibration, of an essential oil is stabilized by the devic forces associated with mother plant, flower, root, or bark. Devic forces are elemental energies or spirits of a plant, which are responsible for holding the blueprint, or the design, for which the plant will be used. On this blueprint is recorded the color of the leaves, the height, the chemical components, the flowers (if any), the innate knowledge of whether the main part of the plant is aboveground or belowground, and much more. So beyond its physiological effects, the energy of the plant offers a multitude of gifts you will uncover in this book. The devic forces of the plant kingdom are wide and varied. The personality and traits of each plant, flower, bush, vine, tree, and so on, are unique. In fact, they are as individual as each one of us.

The energy as maintained by the devic force of the plant brings energy and assistance to humans. Be it the color, shape, size, or the chemical components, these allies assist you on an energetic level. Sure, it might smell yummy and the joy that the olfactory experience brings is part of the shift of consciousness for the better, but its energetic signature goes beyond the extraction of the oil to align us on all levels.

How to Use Essential Oils

There are many ways for essential oils to have positive effects on the body, mind, and spirit. Throughout this book, you will discover oils for almost every use imaginable. The three ways I recommend using essential oils, whether as single notes or part of a blend, are:

1. Diffusion—cold-water mist from a diffuser or mister into the air.

2. Inhalation—smelling the oil or blend directly from the bottle or as a mist.

3. Topically—application to the skin (usually the soles of the feet) with the use of a carrier oil or lotion.

Cautions: Specific Safety Rules for Common Uses

I do not recommend or endorse the internal use of essential oils. The uses described within these pages include inhalation and topical use only. Most oils should not be used during pregnancy or nursing, all are generally contraindicated for the first trimester or nursing, and many should not be used on children under the age of six. For ages six and under, the safest dilution ration is 0.25% dilution, and for over age six, the typical dilution is 1%. For example, if you were to use 6 drops of essential oil in 20 ml of a carrier oil for an adult, then for a child over age six, you would use 1 drop to 100 ml of carrier oil.

Always practice essential oil safety, and remember to use the essential oil in a carrier when applying it to your skin. Any oils that have gone rancid should be discarded. Check on the contraindications in the "For your safety" section under each essential oil to ensure you have a pleasant experience. For instance, some oils lower your blood pressure—like clary sage, sweet marjoram, and ylang-ylang—which may be beneficial for those with high blood pressure but may be harmful for those with low blood pressure.

Common Carrier Oils for Topical Use

If you are planning to use an essential oil topically, it is highly recommended that you use carrier oil. Just as the name implies, carrier oil *carries*, or dilutes, the highly concentrated essential oil for the purposes of application on the body. Carrier oils are oils extracted from nuts, seeds, or vegetables. When you add an essential oil to a carrier oil, the shelf life is significantly and immediately altered, as the oils extracted from nuts, seeds, and vegetables have a shorter shelf life than essential oils do. Incidentally, citrus oils maintain their shelf life best when refrigerated, and all other essential oils should be stored in a cool, dark place. There are many factors that affect the shelf life of oils. See the information about the Shelf Life of Essential Oils later in this chapter.

When choosing a carrier oil for your topical application of an essential oil or essential oil blend, choose from among the following:

- **Sweet almond oil** is derived from the almond nut, which is rich in antioxidants and high in vitamin E. Sweet almond oil is most popular for use as a carrier for essential oils. It is well received by most skin types. It improves the complexion, soothes irritations, and moisturizes and nourishes the skin, leaving it smooth and soft. Sweet almond oil has a clear, pale yellow color and a slightly sweet, nutty scent.

- **Coconut oil,** extracted from the meat of the coconut, is an excellent moisturizer. Coconut oil easily penetrates the skin and is a favorite among massage therapists and medical professionals as a carrier of essential oils. Fractionated coconut oil is claimed not to go rancid. Other advantages of fractionated coconut oil include that it is odorless, colorless, and washes out of fabrics and therefore does not leave a stain. Fractionated coconut oil remains liquid and clear, while the non-fractionated type solidifies at room temperature.

- **Grapefruit seed carrier oil** is pressed from the seeds of the grapefruit. This is not the same as grapefruit essential oil or grapefruit seed extract. The consistency of grapefruit seed carrier oil is similar to canola oil. It has no scent. With its high vitamin C content, this carrier oil aids in healing acne and tones the skin. Due to its astringent nature, it helps clear congestion in the skin. Grapefruit seed carrier oil is virtually colorless and has little or no scent.

- **Jojoba carrier oil** is extracted from the seed of the jojoba bush. This oil is rich in vitamin E and encourages a glowing complexion. It quickly penetrates the skin. Its skin-smoothing and softening effect makes it a great makeup base. It has even been shown to reduce the appearance of pore size with use over time. Jojoba carrier oil has a slight odor and is pale golden yellow to orange in color.

- **Olive oil** has been used for centuries as a skin moisturizer. This benefit results from its high content of linoleic acid (a polyunsaturated fatty acid) as well as its high mineral and vitamin count. The oil is soothing and healing for the skin. Olive oil ranges from yellow to brown to green in color. It does have a distinct odor. Any type of olive oil will serve the intended purpose.

- **Unscented organic lotion**, which is usually made with organic oil and a natural thickening agent, in a pump dispenser bottle is my personal favorite for applying essential oils topically. A good-quality organic lotion will contain at least 80% organic ingredients and is ready-to-use for all skin types. It may contain a variety of oils like coconut oil, sunflower seed oil, shea butter, and apricot kernel oil.

To use a carrier oil or unscented lotion, the essential oil can be added to the bottle itself or a separate glass container for blending, or a portion of the carrier oil can be poured into the palm of your hand along with a few drops of the desired essential oil(s).

Each of the carrier oils just listed are great for use by massage therapists, but for my home personal use, I prefer to use unscented lotion. I simply pump a few dollops of lotion into the palm of my hand, add a few drops of the essential oil(s), then emulsify the mixture in the palms of my hands, and apply it to the soles of my feet.

Essential oil in a carrier, whether oil or lotion, can also be applied to an affected area. However, be sure you are aware of any contraindications. For instance, citrus oils are phototoxic, so when using this particular oil on an exposed part of your body, be mindful to stay out of direct sunlight for a number of hours after application. See the "For your safety" sections in the A-to-Z guide for general contraindications to each oil. It is always best to talk with your healthcare practitioner if you have any medical conditions or concerns and to do further research on any contradictions specific to your ailment.

The Grades of Essential Oils

Aromatherapy products have entered the commercial marketplace by force. There are many commercial-grade products marketed as "aromatherapy," but they are either not made with quality essential oils or contain synthetic fragrances and other impurities. Keep in mind that some essential oils with beneficial properties may have a bit of an unpleasant scent. (These won't typically get shelf space in the commercial-grade air-freshener aisle!) If you plan to use essential oils therapeutically, it is necessary to know and understand the differences between the various grades of essential oils.

True medical-grade oils provide real therapeutic results. They bring about a physiological, mental, emotional, or spiritual response immediately. With the exception of a few resinous oils such as benzoin and patchouli, they are not greasy on your skin. True medical-grade essential oils have the longest shelf life when properly stored in a cool, dark place. Keep in mind that citrus oils are best kept in the refrigerator. Do not leave any oils in extreme heat or cold.

The following is an overview of the various grades of oils you will encounter on the market:

- **Pure Medical Grade/Therapeutic Grade** essential oils are 100% pure and completely natural. This means they do not contain any synthetic or unnatural adulterations. They are determined to be pure through quality control from the point of growth, processing, and laboratory analysis.

- **Pure Grade Organic** essential oils are from organic flowers, plants, and trees that are certified by U.S. standards and inspections. They are considered pure medical grade oils.

- **Aromatherapy Grade** essential oils are adulterated with natural and unnatural components and additives.

- **Commercial Grade** essential oils have been distilled again, creating a lower-grade oil, or have components added or removed to improve odor or safety.

I use medical grade oils for therapeutic reasons. Being the largest organ of the body, the skin is the key location for the absorption of the essential oils directly into the bloodstream. To use therapeutically, add the chosen oil or synergy to carrier oil, as described earlier, and apply it to the soles of your feet to maximize the integration of the oil's physiological benefits. Application to the feet also avoids sensitivity challenges in those with sensitive skin; irritation is less likely to affect the soles of the feet, which are generally thicker-skinned than the rest of the body.

Shelf Life of Essential Oils

It is difficult to predict the shelf life of essential oils. Many external factors can influence the integrity of essential oils. The truth is that anything that interferes with the chemical stability of the oils can cause a process of oxidation or deterioration. Temperature, light, and air can have an effect on the chemical components. Overall, medical-grade or therapeutic-quality essential oils will last longer, depending on the specific oil and conditions of storage. Even under ideal conditions it is hard to predict the deterioration rate.

Some factors that can maintain the freshness of the oils is to keep them stored in a cool, dark place away from direct sunlight and variation in temperatures. Avoid leaving them in your car or on a windowsill where they will be affected by light and temperature changes. The dark-colored glass bottles do offer some protection, yet leaving any oil in heat or in sunlight will contribute to oxidation and deterioration of the essential oil.

According to aromatherapy expert Robert Tisserand, the clock starts when you first open the essential oil and a full, unused bottle will remain fresh for a long time. Here are the guidelines Tisserand provides for essential oils that are refrigerated at 35–38°:

- 1–2 years citrus, frankincense, lemongrass, neroli, pine, spruce, and tea tree

- 2–3 years almost every other essential oil

- 4–8 years patchouli, sandalwood, vetiver

Essential Oil Extraction Methods

Essential oils are derived from various parts of plants including barks, bulbs, dried flower buds, flowers, fruits, grasses, gums, leaves, rhizomes, roots, seeds, tree blossoms, and woods. Most essential oils are extracted through steam distillation, a modern version of hydrodistillation. The extraction method is generally chosen based on which method will bring about the best result for the part of the plant used.

In the A-to-Z section of this book, the part of the plant used for extraction is included in the listing. For example, myrrh is from bark, lemongrass from leaves of the grass, vetiver from root, celery seed from seed, and cedar from wood. This information adds another layer to understanding the energetic vibration of the essential oil. For example, in vibrational healing work, an essential oil that is derived from the root or the wood indicates a stable and grounded energy, whereas an essential oil that is derived from a flower will provide an uplifting, joyful energy. Another example is an essential oil derived from the rind of a citrus fruit, offering support for improved integration of life circumstances.

The following is an overview of the various extraction methods used to extract the essential oil with the chemical components intact.

- **Cold-pressed method** is primarily used to extract the oils of citrus from the peel or rind of the fruit. It is specifically beneficial for citrus extraction, such as orange, lemon, and bergamot, because these volatile oils will oxidize in heat and degrade the medicinal qualities of the oil. (As mentioned, citrus oils are best kept in the refrigerator to maintain the integrity of the oil.)

- **Enfleurage method** is a traditional method of extraction typically used to absorb the aromatic essence from the highest-quality and most delicate flowers such as rose and jasmine. The end product is called an absolute. Because the process is extremely labor-intensive and highly concentrated, these absolutes are more expensive. Using hundreds of petals from the given flower, the essence is absorbed into lard, fat, or olive oil on tiered sheets of glass. The glass is coated with the oil or fat, the petals are sprinkled onto the fat, and then the essence from the petals is absorbed. The resulting pomade (a thick ointment-like substance) is diluted with alcohol and shaken for 24 hours to separate the fat from the essential oil.

- **Solvent extraction** is a process in which immiscible liquids, meaning liquids that cannot be mixed, are vigorously shaken to partition, or separate, the compounds in two different liquids in order to transfer the solutes (the dissolved substance) from one solvent to the other. Alcohol and other solvents may be used on some plant parts, usually flowers, to release the essential oil in a multistep process.

- **Steam distillation** is the use of steam from boiling water to extract the essential oil from the plant. A still, like those used by old-time moonshiners, is used, allowing the water to pass through plant material to produce a steam that travels through cooled coils. The volatile essence floats to the top of the water and is removed.

Aromatic Notes in Essential Oils

Blending essential oils to create a fragrant blend is both an art and a science. Essential oils are generally categorized into basic groups, such as camphorous, citrus, earthy, floral, herbaceous, medicinal, spicy, and woodsy, to name a few. As you become familiar with these basic groups and the associated essential oils, you will find this information beneficial when creating a blend. For example, if you want to make the blend sweeter, you would add a floral scent; if you want to make the scent more stable, you would add an earthy oil.

Essential oils can also be categorized using the analogy of the musical scale, which loosely corresponds with the above groups. For example, floral oils are generally top notes; earthy and woodsy oils are generally base notes; herbaceous oils are typically middle-to-top notes; and camphorous, citrusy, and medicinal oils are often middle notes. Generally speaking, top notes evaporate in 1–2 hours, middle notes may last 2–4 hours, and base notes can take days to evaporate. Base notes are also used to stabilize the volatility of a blend.

- **Top notes** are the fastest-acting and the quickest to evaporate. They are stimulating and uplifting to mind and body. Top notes often have antiviral properties. These oils include basil, bergamot, cinnamon, clary sage, eucalyptus, grapefruit, lemon, lemongrass, lime, neroli, niaouli, orange, peppermint, petitgrain, ravensara, sage, tea tree, and thyme.

- **Middle notes** primarily affect the general metabolism and physical functions of the body and have a balancing effect. The majority of essential oils are middle notes. These oils include cardamom, chamomile, cypress, fennel, geranium, juniper berry, lavender, melissa, pine, and spikenard.

- **Base notes** are heavier oils in that they actually weigh more in measurement by ounces and pounds and are often thicker than top notes and middle notes. For instance, an 8-ounce bottle of vetiver, which is a base note, will have what *appears* to be less oil than an 8-ounce bottle of lavender, which is a thinner oil. Base notes are the slowest to evaporate. They are also the most sedative and relaxing of the oils. Base note oils are considered fixatives, meaning they slow down the evaporation (balance the volatility) of other oils within a blend. Base notes include cedarwood, cinnamon, clove, frankincense, ginger, jasmine, myrrh, patchouli, rose, rosewood, sandalwood, vetiver, and ylang-ylang.

As you start to work and play with essential oils, begin by getting to know single notes—that is, one essential oil at a time. Just as you get to know your friends, you will get to know each of the oils and what they can do and how they make you feel on all levels—spiritually, mentally, emotionally, and physically. Eventually you will come to understand and feel which essential oils will work well together for different purposes. Using the analogy of friends, as you become well acquainted with each, you know how everyone will get along and when to include them in a gathering for the best results.

Recommendation for Beginner's Use

I recommend inhalation and diffusion as the preferred methods of use until you get to know your essential oil allies a little better. Always remember that essential oils have true chemical constituents with real effects on your body. Medical grade essential oils are much more potent than a roll-on fragranced oil. So use them sparingly, as a little bit goes a long way. Once you know a particular oil well, you can then graduate to the next level by applying the essential oil in a carrier oil to the soles of your feet. Refrain from applying the oils directly on your body and do not take them internally. Other than that, have a good time exploring the many uses of nature's aromatic gifts and turn to the myriad of vibrational supports available to you as you begin creating aroma-energetic blends with far-reaching beneficial effects.

CHAPTER TWO

• •

Vibrational Assistance for Your Aroma-Energetic Practices

Everything holds a vibration, has a vibrational signature, and emanates energy. A vibration is the energetic frequency, or atmosphere, associated with a person, animal, place, or thing. It is something that can be felt and communicated energetically. We have established that this is true for the energy of people, places, situations, flowers, food, animals, gardens, homes, and so on, and as I discuss in my book *The Essential Guide to Crystals, Minerals and Stones,* it is also true for those precious gifts from nature. The elements found in the A-to-Z section of the following pages include essential oils, flower essences, gemstone essences, holy water, divine messengers, the chakra system, the zodiac, planets, numbers, and animals.

Everything that is created, including our individual lives, is manifested through the intention of our thoughts, actions, words, and deeds. Our intentions vibrate out into the world and return to us in the form of our personal reality. Therefore, to create the life you want, your focus must be on what you do want, not on what you don't want. Whatever you focus on becomes your reality. In other words, all of your conscious thoughts and feelings—as well as the subconscious and unconscious ones—create the life you are currently living. This basic principle is at the heart of most universal laws, including the law of attraction and the laws of physics.

In this section, you'll learn about various sources of vibrational support as you set the intention to make the changes you want to see in your life. For example, flower essences—"vibrational medicine"—can be used to provide balance by realigning the emotional and mental bodies. When used in conjunction with essential oils, flower essences provide a higher and deeper component to balance body, mind, and spirit on an energetic level. Meanwhile, chakra awareness through the understanding of the associated qualities for each of these energy centers provides yet another recalibration tool. Chakra rebalancing is more complete when the olfactory nerve plays a part as a reminder to stay focused on the intended goal.

Gemstone essences are excellent additions to aromatic-energetic blends to raise the vibration of the synergy. The gemstone kingdom brings color and geometric vibrational healing to the mix. You can add these essences, which you will learn how to create later in the book, to a blend just as you would do with flower essences to help maintain and amplify your focus on the intended positive results.

Each of the discussions to follow provides more detail about these vibrational tools to familiarize you with how they can enhance your healing and transformation as part of your aromatherapeutic practices.

Flower Essences

Throughout the A-to-Z guide, listed with each essential oil, you will see references to flower essences and the associated energetic connections for bringing about balance on a mental and emotional level. Flower essences are vibrational preparations used for specific purposes. Unlike essential oils, they do not contain the chemical components extracted from the plant, bark, root, and so on. Instead, flower essences are derived from the energetic vibration of the plant, tree, or flower. The healing provided is through the use of intention to realign the emotional and mental bodies. Although I do not recommend the ingestion of essential oils, flower essences are meant to be taken internally. While there are many producers of flower essence collections, the ones referred to within this book are the Bach Flower Remedies. You can purchase Bach Flower Remedies at natural grocery stores, health food and vitamin stores, and some metaphysical stores and holistic centers.

The developer of Bach Flower Remedies, Dr. Edward Bach, was a successful bacteriologist and homeopathic physician. At a young age, he dreamed of finding a cure for all diseases. He knew that the out-of-balance conditions of the body stemmed from mental and emotional challenges—negative thoughts and feelings. He gave up his lucrative practice in search of a gentle method of healing to realign the emotional body, which naturally corrects an issue with the physical body. In the 1930s, Dr. Bach discovered these gentle energetic vibrational essences, which are now used all over the world. Dr. Edward Bach wrote in his book *The Bach Flower Remedies*, "Disease of the body itself is nothing but the result of the disharmony between soul and mind. Remove the disharmony, and we regain harmony between soul and mind, and the body is once more perfect in all its parts."

The Bach Flower Remedies are intended to transform negative attitudes or beliefs into positive ones, thereby allowing the body's own physical system to fight disease and the stress associated with an out-of-balance condition.

The use of Bach Flower Remedies requires no training; all that is required is the ability to understand oneself or another on a mental and emotional level. I recommend that people discover for themselves which essence is best for them, rather than go to someone else to tell them what they need. Pamphlets, brochures, and other guides help you determine which essence or series of essences are best for you in this moment. There are thirty-eight Bach Flower Remedies, each of which is associated with various feelings. Use flower essences during challenging times when negative feelings arise, or when you are feeling exhaustion, with the intention to restore balance before physical symptoms show up.

I have personally used Bach Flower Remedies for over twenty years with great results. These energetic treasures helped me through the release of a cigarette habit, relationship ups and downs, high anxiety during the aftermath of the September 11th disaster, the death of my parents, premenstrual syndrome, menopause, moving, and stock market cycles.

The directions for usage vary depending on which of the company's pamphlets you are reviewing, but they all provide appropriate guidelines. One pamphlet says to place 2 drops directly on your tongue and to add 4 drops to your water at least 4 times a day. Others say to add 2 drops to water or juice. Another pamphlet recommends creating a blend in an amber dropper bottle filled three-quarters of the way with spring water by adding 2 drops of each essence, which you would then take 4 drops of 4 times a day, especially upon rising and just before bed.

It is generally established that you should continue to use the selected essences for the given issue until you realize that a shift has taken place inside you and you are over the issue(s) that initiated your desire to take the essences in the first place.

While there varying opinions about exactly how to use Bach Flower Essences, I have successfully used them as follows:

I review the list of feelings/situations associated with each of the thirty-eight essences and assign a number from 1 to 10 to each one. A 10 indicates that I feel a certain essence most describes me or how I am feeling. Depending on my needs, I choose from two to six essences to achieve balance.

I add one drop of each essence to my first 16- to 20-ounce glass of water in the morning and, when I think about it, to the subsequent glasses I drink throughout the day. If my stress levels are particularly high, I make sure to add it every time I fill another glass or bottle.

I sometimes add the essences to my bathwater along with the complementary essential oils. With just a drop or two, the flower essences actually change the energetics of the bathwater. I also add the essences to the combination of gemstone essences, holy water, and sacred site essences to create The Crystal Garden's aroma-energetic blends. To do this, I use a sterilized jar with a lid as the container. I add the following ingredients: distilled water, grain alcohol, the specific gemstones needed for the given intention, Bach Flower Remedies for the specific intention, holy waters, sacred site essences, and other sacred waters collected from rivers, streams, and springs. These combinations are utilized in quantities of less than 1 ml per 16 ounces of distilled water. The energetic water combination of sacred waters is added to the essential oil blends for external use. After about 24 hours, the vibrational synergy is ready to add to an aromatherapy blend that is intended to be sprayed on and around the body through a mister. This vibrational synergy and essential oils are for external use only. Do not ingest this combination because there is no way to establish the cleanliness of water collected from rivers, streams, and springs.

See Appendix B for choosing the best Bach Flower Remedies for your synergistic blends as well as single remedies for traditional use.

Gemstone Essences

Throughout the A-to-Z guide, listed with each essential oil, you will see a corresponding gemstone, mineral, or crystal. Like everything in our world, gemstones, minerals, and crystals have a vibrational signature, which can assist us in rebalancing and realigning energetically and physically. When you add the vibrational essences of gemstones to your synergistic mix, you amplify the vibration and potential for healing, focus, and balance.

In my work with scents, colors, and crystals over the past thirty years, I've found that to use any vibrational tool most effectively it is best to associate an intention with it. The more information you have about the qualities associated with certain stones and how they correspond to the oils, colors, essences, and so on, the more creative you can be when using these valuable tools to create your intentions and improve your life.

In this book, I am introducing the use of crystals or gems as vibrational essences. Just as Edward Bach and other flower essence aficionados have created essences using the vibration emanating from a flower, I do the same using gemstones, and you can do this easily as well. (See the directions for making gemstone essences below.) A great way to use the gemstone essence is to combine it with your chosen essential oils and other essences to amplify and accent the intention of your aroma-energetic blend.

Creating aroma-energetic sprays and mists is a creative way to refocus your mental, physical, spiritual, and emotional bodies back to an aligned state of being. There is no limit to creating and using combinations of the energetic vibrations to help you maintain focus on what you do want versus what you don't want. As you use these gemstone essences in combination with an aromatherapy blend and flower essences, use the affirmation combined with your intention to transform your reality.

Caution: DO NOT ingest gemstone essences. Do not drink any water that has had rocks or crystals soaking in it, as unknown and potentially poisonous minerals can leech out of the stone into the water.

How to Make a Gemstone Essence

To make a gemstone essence, decide on the purpose of the essence. To help determine your gemstone essence formula, use the A-to-Z guide and the appendices for guidance and inspiration. Begin with questions such as, "What are my goals? How do I want the combination to help me?" Once you have identified your intention, choose the gemstones that match. The A-to-Z guide and the gemstone combination recommendations in Appendix C for common goals and intentions will help you get started.

Once you have gathered your chosen stones, you will also need the following supplies:

- Glass jar with a lid
- 151-proof grain alcohol or your choice of high-proof liquor
- Distilled water
- Clear focus and intention
- Label

Gently place the stones into the jar, maintaining your focus on the reason you are putting this combination together. Cover the stones with distilled water. Fill the jar about three-quarters of the way. Add approximately 1 to 2 ounces of grain alcohol to stabilize the energetics, or vibrational essence, of the combination. Put the lid on the jar. Wipe the jar with a towel to dry off any moisture. Create a label listing not only the contents of the jar (that is, the stones and liquids), but also and most important, your intention for the gemstone essence. Adhere the label to the jar.

The various combinations of gemstones are virtually unlimited. In Appendix C you will find a few sample combinations of stones and suggested affirmations to create your gemstone essences, along with a corresponding archangel. (See the section "Divine Messengers" later in this chapter for more on the archangels.)

Holy Water

Water, by nature, is a cleansing, nourishing, and integral part of life here on this planet. Throughout history, water has been associated with spiritual cleansing and blessings. The term *holy water* generally indicates that the water has been blessed by a member of the clergy or religious figure for use in blessings or cleansing. After apprenticing with a medicine man and traveling to various sacred sites many years ago, my definition of holy water became a bit broader and more inclusive. Holy water is water that has been prayed over or transformed through intention, contemplation, and meditation. Adding holy water to your essential oil blends adds another level of energy and vibrational assistance to synergetic blends, thereby creating an important aroma-energetic tool.

I grew up blessed with a wonderful mother whose range of spiritual and metaphysical intuition was extraordinary. It took me many years after her passing to recognize the magnitude of her profound spiritual connection and wisdom. In our household, it was custom to be blessed with holy water or oil. Sometimes it was to help us heal from an illness, but other times, I now realize, it was to maintain a protective circle around our family.

I have traveled to many parts of the world. At almost every church I've been to, I have collected holy water. If the church was old or not often used, the holy water font was sometimes dry. That is when I had the idea to create my own holy water. The first time I did this was during a spiritual adventure when I visited the Chapelle Saint-Germain de Cesseras located in Languedoc-Roussillon in southern France.

I filled an amber bottle with drinking water and placed within it a few tiny clear quartz crystals. I left the cap off during a meditation and toning session. (Toning is a song-like vocalization of extended notes for rebalancing oneself on all levels.) I focused my intention that all the good energy from our experience in that beautiful chapel would be captured energetically within the waters of that bottle.

When the session was over, I knew that the vibrational essence of the sacred space was transmitted into the water through intention and sound waves. I capped the bottle and now use these holy waters in small amounts in vibrational essence formulas. One drop of the holy water in distilled water with grain alcohol will increase the power and effect. The vibrational frequency combined with the intention to capture the energy of the space changes the structure and vibration of the water that was originally placed in the bottle. Masaru Emoto, a Japanese researcher, showed that human consciousness has an effect on the molecular structure of water. Along the same lines, the combination of the energetic vibration of the sacred space and the intention I held when making the sacred site essence created the vibrational essence.

I've also created holy water simply by forming an intention to purify and sanctify the water and placing my hands over the glass container or bowl. (I use distilled water for this purpose.) Sometimes I also pray aloud over the water. When I create holy water, I always focus on transferring and preserving the energy of love and well-being into the water. Sometimes I feel the energy passing through the palms of my hands and infusing the water with blessings and love. Anyone can do this by forming a positive intention.

Water is a wonderful way to cleanse not only ourselves but also our minds and hearts. With the right intention, even a swimming pool can become a holy body of water. I often pray while swimming and exercising in my backyard pool. I maintain my focus on specific people, places, or situations that need healing, love, or support. I also find it joyful to maintain focus on the many blessings in my life, so I do much of my gratitude contemplation in my pool as well. By the time I step out of the pool, I perceive that the whole pool—all that water—has become holy water. I enjoyed recently discovering that bathing in holy water is a key practice in Hinduism, and the Ganges River is considered the holiest river by the Hindus. While my backyard pool certainly isn't the Ganges River, I do feel blessed having made my pool experience a holy one.

Knowing my love for the energetics that holy waters offer, many friends, colleagues, and acquaintances have gifted me with holy water from rivers, sacred sites, cathedrals, and the like. Holy water from various sources has become an integral ingredient in my own line of aroma-energetic sprays. You can also use holy water for this purpose and create your own blends.

Many people are familiar with the concept of baptism with water or entering a Catholic church and dipping your fingers into the font of holy water to bless yourself. While the water itself doesn't contain magical properties, the power of the water is contained within the prayers and faith of the individual using the holy water. The intention installed on a vibrational level makes this water sacred. Buddhist shrines usually have a water vessel within their walls. I personally observed H.H. Dalai Lama sprinkling water from a vessel with a peacock feather during a Kalachakra initiation. Temple tanks containing water in Hindu temples are believed to be holy and have cleansing properties. The integration of water in most Hindu rituals is used for spiritual cleansing.

St. Theresa of Avila, a patron saint of writers and a writer herself, was a prominent Spanish mystic and a strong believer in holy water to repel evil and negativity. Holy water's use to repel evil influences is widespread in literature involving mythical creatures and vampires. Even Dorothy from *The Wizard of Oz* used water to defeat the Wicked Witch. And as you know, there is always some truth in fiction.

Holy water can be used for clearing away real or imagined entity attachments to relieve a person of disturbing symptoms associated with such attachments. An entity attachment is a fear-based energy created through one's personal fears or belief in the influence of a lower-level energy such as a dark force or disincarnate spirit. These energies can weaken your energetic field as well as your ability to deal with life in a positive way. Keep in mind that an entity attachment can be real or imagined, as I mentioned in the beginning of this paragraph. A person may simply believe he or she is cursed or that there is an otherworldly attachment in their energetic field. Most cases I've encountered are actually an accumulation of negative vibrations stored in a person's energy field as a result of erroneous personal beliefs, negative self-talk, engrained self-doubt, and fears. Some entity attachments, however, can very well arise from others who prey on a person's vulnerable nature.

In this book, holy water is an ingredient used to raise the vibration or energetic essence of your aromatherapy practice. The holy water adds blessings and love to shift your energetic field and ultimately balance your spiritual, mental, emotional, and physical body. Using holy water along with the essential oils and other complementary vibrational tools shared throughout this book helps to restore balance and maintain a flow of positive energy and blessings in your life.

An excellent way to release negativity and replace it with positive intentions is to anoint yourself with holy water by pouring it over your body following a shower. Use a combination of distilled water, holy water, essential oil, Bach Flower Remedy, gemstone essences, and a positive intention to create your sacred blend. It is most beneficial to anoint yourself for seven to ten consecutive days immediately following your morning shower. During this period, it is a must to also use only clean clothes, towels, and bed linens. The combination of cleanliness, prayer, and an aroma-energetic sacred blend creates an energetic vibration that signals the Universe and your Higher Self that you reject anything that is no longer for your highest good.

To perform this ritual, use a metal or glass mixing bowl or a large measuring cup filled with warm water. Place your choice of aromatic essences into the water. One cup at a time, pour the holy water over your body in the following order, while saying a prayer as you pour it: 1) head, 2) heart/left side of body, 3) liver/right side of body, and 4) back of neck. Use the following prayer or write your own with similar sentiments:

———

As a child of God and the Universe, I release any negativity that has been tied to my soul and my spirit. In the name of the Divine Creator, whom I love with all my heart, my soul, and my senses, I command that all the spirits and negative energies that do not belong to me leave my body now. I invoke the high spirits of Adonai, Elohim, and Jehovah whose presence I ask to be with me in

this moment. I invoke the protection and Love of Archangel Michael. Thank you for the all blessings I have in my life.

Adonai, Elohim, and Jehovah are all Hebrew names for God, and hold a strong vibration when petitioning for assistance from the heavenly realm.

Sacred Spiritual Scents for Divine Alignment

Scent is invisible but perceptible. It plays an important role in our spiritual practices, religious ceremonies, and connection with the Divine and the part of us that often remains hidden. Fragrance and scent add varying levels and dimensions to our spiritual states of consciousness. The scent of flowers, fragrance, anointing oils, resins, and incense help to bring about transcendent experiences by way of the olfactory nerve (which carries the sensory information for our sense of smell) and the brain's limbic system (which supports various functions, including our emotions). Sacred spiritual scents align us with greater potential for self-actualization and alignment with angels, saints, Ascended Masters, and loved ones on the other side. (Ascended Masters are highly evolved souls who serve humanity for the fulfillment of personal soul contracts and development as well as planetary well-being.)

Certain scents are associated with various spiritual archetypes. For example, the scent of roses is often associated with Mother Mary, or the Divine Feminine. Saint Therese of Lisieux, known as the Little Flower, is associated with lilies, orris root, jasmine, violets, and roses. Her signature is the rose, which is her way of sending a sign to anyone who needs to know his or her prayers have been heard. In 1531, Our Lady of Guadalupe proved her identity to Juan Diego, an Aztec Indian, with Castilian roses growing on the dry dessert hill on which she had appeared. These are just a few of the examples of the spiritual realm providing signs through scent.

Modern-day saint Sathya Sai Baba (1926–2011), an Indian guru and spiritual teacher, was believed to be a reincarnation of Sai Baba of Shirdi, who died in 1918. You might know the scent associated with Sai Baba as the smell that permeates most New Age and metaphysical stores. Nag Champa incense and oil is enjoyed by millions. Its primary scent comes from the champaca flower from the Magnolia champaca tree, Halmaddi from the Ailanthus malabarica tree, and sandalwood, along with other resins and herbs. Champaca is often found on sacred grounds of Hindu temples or ashrams in connection with the Hindu deity Vishnu. It is used to aid in spiritual connection and meditation.

Scented smoke has been part of spiritual ceremonies for centuries. Certain incenses or resins activate a sense of heightened awareness. They are burned to enliven a part of our consciousness for the purposes of divination and seeking higher wisdom and knowledge. Burning sage and other herbs through the process of smudging, or cleansing, an area releases negative energies. In fact, white sage is well known in metaphysical communities today for clearing away negativity and bad influences and replacing them with love and well-being. Copal and other resins are used in native Mexican fire ceremonies to activate the connection with Great Spirit, while frankincense and myrrh amplify the spiritual connection and cleanse the space in Catholic rituals.

The use of smoke and smudge for shamanic work has been used historically by indigenous cultures worldwide, providing the practitioner with a stronger Divine connection to perform his or her work as a healer, teacher, and divinatory guide. This scented smoke also offers a sacred vibration to the participants in a shamanic circle who are attending the healings or ceremonies. North American Indians used hogweed, red elder bark, and juniper berries in their smudging formulas. The North American Kiowa used sweetgrass as incense, the Cheyenne used it for purification and to ward off evil, Blackfoot and Sioux used it to purify, and all of these and other Native American tribes used it for protection and blessings.

For many years, I burned my own blend of herbs, including sage, cedar, frankincense, copal, dragon's blood, palo santo, sahumerio, osha root, lavender buds, and sandalwood powder, at the beginning of every sacred circle gathering to invite and invoke the wisdom of the ancestors, angels, spirit guides, and Ascended Masters. Eventually, I switched out the smoky version with aroma-energetic Smudge in Spray, for the respiratory well-being of all the participants. An aroma-energetic mist or spray is a liquid alternative to burning herbs. In my aroma-energetic blends, I also include gemstone essences, Bach

Flower Remedies, sacred site essences, and holy water—each of which you will learn about in this book. This vibrational assistance gives the blends an even higher energetic level.

Divine Messengers

You will find archangels, Ascended Masters, and saints referenced throughout the A-to-Z guide as well as in other sections of this book. Call upon this entourage of spirit guides and guardians when you are creating and using your blends. Because humans have free will, angels need to be asked to assist us or intervene on our behalf.

Whether you are conscious of them or not, you have *many* invisible helpers around you at every moment of your life. Imagine them or just know there is a large group of invisible helpers ready to come to your aid. They're watching over you, inspiring you, and guiding you on your path through life. They're with you 24/7, whether you are sleeping or awake. And they're just a thought away when you're ready to be conscious of them. Angels, Ascended Masters, and saints from many spiritual traditions have a vibration and provide energetic assistance to us upon request.

The personalities and qualities of these spiritual beings bring a plethora of positive vibes to your spiritual table. The legions of angels and archangels provide a mystical connection relating to the essential oils in the A-to-Z guide. Whether it is an archangel or an Ascended Master, recognize that these beings of love, light, and well-being can easily become part of your spiritual entourage as you navigate your life during your time here on this planet.

Archangels are messenger angels of high rank. They are beings of love and light with designated responsibilities to guide and assist us here on Earth. Despite their masculine- or feminine-sounding names, they are androgynous light beings without gender, available to help us when invoked or petitioned for a specific purpose in alignment with the Divine plan. Align with Archangel Michael every day and night until it is an automatic habit. Visualize and imagine Archangel Michael before you, Archangel Raphael behind you, Archangel Gabriel on your left side, Archangel Uriel on your right side, and your Guardian Angel above you. Don't worry too much about who is where, but do invite all five of those angels to aid you in changing and shifting your reality to one of inner peace, harmony, and love. Imagine a strong connection of roots of white light from the soles of your feet into the ever-loving Mother Earth. Know and believe you are Divinely protected.

You will find additional information in Appendix D regarding the angels, Ascended Masters, and saints.

Chakra System

Throughout the A-to-Z guide, listed with each essential oil, you will see the corresponding chakra(s). The word *chakra* is a Sanskrit word for "wheel" or "vortex." Understanding the chakras is just one of many avenues to increase your personal power and awareness and enhance the vibration of your aromatic-energetic blends through intention and visualization.

You have seven chakras, all of which are energetically interconnected within the subtle bodies, which comprise your thoughts (mental body), your feelings (emotional body), and your connection with spirit (spiritual body). Within all four bodies, there are seven chakras—the crown, the third eye, the throat, the heart, the solar plexus, the navel, and the root—each associated with a specific color.

The first chakra is the root chakra. Its basic color is red. This energy center is located at the base of the spine and is responsible for our basic needs. This is where we store our vital energy for providing food, shelter, and water for ourselves. It is the base of Maslow's pyramid. These are our very basic needs, and money is strongly associated with this center.

The second chakra is the navel or sacral chakra. Its main color is orange. It is located at the navel. This is the center for reproduction and creativity. We often store emotional memories in this center. It is a center that allows us to create and take action in our lives.

The third chakra is the solar plexus chakra and is located at the solar plexus (the area of the body between your belly button and the center of the chest). The main color associated with this chakra is yellow. This is the place of joy, personal power, self-confidence, mental clarity, and the ability to shine our light. We often store verbal abuses here that may have reduced our self-esteem and likewise store kudos and praises we have received that raised our self-confidence.

The fourth chakra is the heart center. This chakra is green and/or pink. It is located in the center of the chest. This center is the bridge between the lower three chakras of the physical, mundane world and the upper chakras of the spiritual world. This is the part of us where our true self resides ... the Love That We Are. It is where and how we integrate that we are spiritual beings having a physical experience.

The fifth chakra is the throat center. This chakra is blue (like the color of the sky) or turquoise. This center is located at our throat and provides us with our ability to communicate and express ourselves. This is not exclusively our verbal expression but also the way we express ourselves in the world, including writing, speaking, singing, cooking, or however else we may express who and what we are.

The sixth chakra is the third eye center. This chakra is indigo blue. It is located in the center of the forehead. This is the location of our ability to see the unseen, know the unknown, and hear what is not being said. It is the place of intuition, knowing, and dreaming.

The seventh chakra is the crown chakra. The color associated with this chakra ranges from golden white light to a violet flame. This is the place of higher intuition, channeling, and the connection with Divine consciousness. This is the place where our connection to miracles resides.

When one or more of your chakras become blocked or out of alignment, your mental state or your emotional balance is affected. A blocked chakra can also affect you spiritually. Eventually, the blockage presents itself on the physical level in the form of dis-ease or some health condition that seems to show up out of nowhere. However, the block or lack of well-being isn't really out of nowhere. Every thought, action, and intention established the groundwork to present the challenge. Self-awareness and being truly conscious of your thoughts, feelings, and actions can shift your reality and lead you to a deeply positive life experience.

You will find additional information in Appendix D regarding the chakras and which essential oils aid in balancing a specific chakra.

Zodiac, Planets, Numbers, and Animals

Throughout the A-to-Z guide, listed with each essential oil, you will see entries for the corresponding signs of the zodiac, planetary bodies, numbers, and animals.

Each sign of the zodiac and planetary body has certain qualities and traits. Just as there are associated astrological designations for each gemstone, which I included in *The Essential Guide to Crystals, Minerals and Stones*, these associations likewise apply to grasses, flowers, plants, trees, and bushes and the essential oils extracted from them. With a little knowledge of the asteroids, planets, and zodiac signs, you will get to know each essential oil on a deeper level.

Like everything, numbers also have a vibration. Numerology is a metaphysical tool that offers the significance and meanings of numbers and number sequences. Symbolism and synchronicity enrich our lives by providing information about a person's personality and traits. With an understanding of the energy associated with numbers, you can gain deeper knowledge of the strengths, talents, and nature of a person, place, or situation based on the numerological association. An understanding of the meanings of numbers and the vibrations associated with them also offers you another level of understanding of the vibration of a given essential oil. Take the time to investigate the meanings of each number and use that information to familiarize yourself with the energetic vibration as you use them in your aroma-energetic blends.

Animals, birds, insects, reptiles, and sea life have certain qualities and mannerisms that can also be associated with the vibration of an essential oil. The ways these creatures exhibit behaviors and ways of being on this planet bring us lessons and messages for self-awareness and aid in awakening of consciousness. The appearance of animals and other creatures offer another avenue for self-observation. Just as crystals, plants, the zodiac, and numbers carry a vibration, the animals have a vibrational field that support us as allies and guides. By understanding the messages and mannerisms of various animals whose energy enters your life either physically or mentally, you can make necessary adjustments in how you perceive yourself and reality. This concept is associated with Native American spirituality and the spirituality of many indigenous tribes around the world.

Throughout the A-to-Z section, you will find one or more animals, birds, insects, reptiles, and/or sea life listed with each essential oil. This entry provides you an avenue to delve even deeper into the nature of the given essential oil.

———————

People have personified nature in their drawings for centuries. The personification of nature is the attribution of a characteristic, usually associated with a human quality, to something that isn't human, like a plant or animal. Anthropomorphism, another moniker for personification, depicts the forces of nature along with animals and plants in storytelling as a literary device. It is traditionally used in fables and has ancient roots in literature.

In many ways, the associations and cross-associations between plants, animals, angels, gemstones, flowers, and essential oils that you find throughout this book provide a personification or identity that is beyond the physical. It is a metaphysical association to garner a deeper relationship with All That Is. Everything is connected, and all life can provide us with wisdom and knowledge. Plants and animals have spirits and lessons to share with us.

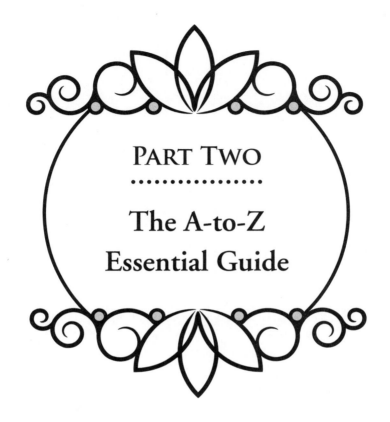

PART TWO

The A-to-Z
Essential Guide

In the pages that follow you will find a directory of essential oils listed in alphabetical order. Each entry includes the following categories:

Essential Oil

Key phrase: A few words that provide quick insight into the specific vibration of the essential oil.

Botanical name: A formal scientific name for the plant from which the oil is derived.

Note: A classification of essential oils originally based on the musical scale. Top, middle, and base notes are used in synergies to create a balanced blend.

Method of extraction: The process used to extract the oil from the plant.

Parts used: The part of the plant used (e.g., flower, bark, root, twigs, or leaf).

Fragrance: A description of the scent or odor of the essential oil.

Color(s): The energetic frequency associated with the colors of the chakras system on a spiritual, mental, emotional, and physical level. The color listed relates to the color associated with the plant from which the oil has been extracted. In some cases the color is related to the color of the oil or the energetic vibrational color that will help restore balance through the use of the essential oil.

Chakra(s): The chakra(s) that benefit most from the essential oil.

Astrological sign(s): The sign of the zodiac with which the oil is associated, based on my thirty years of study with various teachers. (This varies from source to source.)

Planet(s): The planetary body, including asteroids, with which the oil is associated. This may or may not correspond with the astrological sign assigned.

Number(s): The matching numerological vibration based on my knowledge of numerology and/or as a result of Divine inspiration. In some cases, double digits followed by a single digit, separated by a slash, are listed to provide a more complete numerological portrayal of the oil.

Animal(s): The power animal with which the oil is associated, which provides a deeper understanding of the oil's vibrational energy.

Element(s): The element—air, fire, water, metal, or earth—associated with the essential oil. The choice of element included in this entry was determined by either how the plant grows or by the human interaction (that is, how it affects the four subtle bodies).

Affirmation: A positive statement of affirmation associated with the essential oil that helps to focus an intention.

Complementary flower essences: The Bach Flower Essences that support the intention and uses of the essential oil.

Complementary stones: The gemstones that support the intention and uses of the essential oil.

About the plant: A basic description of the plant.

Chemical components: The individual chemical constituents that identify the medicinal properties of the essential oil.

Spiritual uses: Insight on how to use the oil to further develop your spiritual connection. The spiritual use of the oil is the manner in which it can help you develop your spiritual nature or your spiritual practice. Common suggestions are offered regarding connection with the Divine, regression therapy for a better understanding of spiritual lessons, meditation practice, and connection with guides, angels, and other master teachers in a variety of ways.

Mental uses: Insight on how to use the oil for mental focus or clarity as well as situations in which it can be helpful. In some cases, the oil literally affects the central nervous system, and other times, it is the energy of the essential oil that realigns the mind. The mental subtle body contains all the thoughtforms in your consciousness that create your reality. To manage and balance your thoughtforms is paramount in creating a happy, healthy, and productive life. Use the oil with the intention to keep your mind focused on the positive: what you do want, not what you don't want.

Emotional uses: Insight on how to use the oil as a tool for dealing with feelings to unblock underlying challenges. The emotional body is just as real as the physical body. You don't have to be convinced that you have feelings. This entry is dedicated to how the oil can help you get in touch with, embrace, or transform and transmute your feelings. Balance is always the goal, and it starts by understanding and recognizing how you feel.

Physical uses: Insight on how to use the oil to support the physical body and mundane daily existence, including financial security and career support. It refers to the designation of either the physical body or the manner in which you exist. Aromatherapy ally designations regarding professions are included here. (Caution: Do not use the essential oils internally in any way. Do not put essential oils in water you plan to drink.)

Therapeutic properties: A list of all the ways you can use this oil therapeutically.

Divine guidance: Guidance for uncovering self-knowledge and self-realization for the purpose of personal development and spiritual awakening.

For your safety: Contraindications or potential hazards or cautions.

Interesting tidbits. Information about history, lore, or use of the essential oil in perfumery.

ALLSPICE
Gratitude for All That Is

BOTANICAL NAME	*Pimenta dioica*
NOTE	middle
METHOD OF EXTRACTION	steam distillation
PARTS USED	berries
FRAGRANCE	strong and spicy; a mix of clove, cinnamon, and cardamom; reminiscent of Thanksgiving spices
COLOR(S)	brown, gold
CHAKRA(S)	all
ASTROLOGICAL SIGN(S)	Capricorn, Leo
PLANET(S)	Saturn, Sun
NUMBER(S)	88
ANIMAL(S)	eagle, turkey
ELEMENT(S)	fire

Affirmation I am grateful for the abundance and prosperity in my life. I enjoy my loyal and supportive friends and family. Everything I need or want is always available to me. I am a blessing to others as well as myself. Love, wealth, and plentitude come naturally to me. I have many blessings.

Complementary flower essences Elm for temporary exhaustion and feelings of depression. *Hornbeam* for feeling overwhelmed and exhausted. *Oak* to take steps toward rejuvenation.

Complementary stones All gemstones, but especially amazonite, black tourmaline, chalcopyrite, copper, emerald, galena, green aventurine, hematite, pyrite.

About the plant Allspice is an evergreen tree that reaches a height of 30 to 80 feet. It has fragrant leaves and small, white flowers that turn into berries.

Chemical components Eugenol, methyl eugenol, limonene, cineole, phellandrene, terpinolene, caryophyllene, selinene.

Spiritual uses Allspice is one of the scents associated with Archangel Michael. This essential oil is a good addition to meditation blends; it helps to improve the quality of the breath because it opens the breathing passages. Allspice warms the spirit and has a strong affiliation with the Divine Masculine.

Mental uses Allspice helps achieve mental clarity and focus, grounding your thoughts and relaxing the mind enough to sort through ideas. It helps improve mental capacity during times of exhaustion. For most people, allspice brings back pleasant memories of maternal comfort.

Emotional uses Allspice has a comforting scent and offers a sensation of warmth and relaxation during times of emotional stress. The energetic of this oil is suggestive of a strong, positive energy watching over you during challenging life situations. Allspice lifts your spirits when you are feeling down or dejected. Inhale this essential oil while you repeat the affirmations above.

Physical uses Allspice provides a numbing effect on the nerves and therefore relieves pain. The anesthetic quality of allspice is only effective locally; it doesn't affect the central nervous system. It is helpful for joint pain as well as pain resulting from insect bites and stings. Allspice is a good aromatherapy ally for bakers, neurologists, and those in law enforcement.

Therapeutic properties Analgesic, antidepressant, antioxidant, antiseptic, aphrodisiac, astringent, carminative, digestive, relaxant, rubefacient, sedative, stimulative, stomachic, tonic.

Divine guidance Have you been experiencing mental cloudiness? Are you ready to accept prosperity and inner peace into your life? Recognize your inner strength—mental, physical, emotional, and spiritual. There are plenty of people, places, and situations for which you are grateful. Now is the time to put your attention on all that is good.

For your safety Avoid in cases of liver disease and hemophilia; possible irritant to skin and mucous membranes.

> ### Interesting tidbits:
> Allspice is also called Jamaica pepper, myrtle pepper, pimento berry, and pimento. Allspice is an important ingredient in Caribbean jerk seasoning as well as in Bay Rum.

ANGELICA
Hear the Angels Sing

BOTANICAL NAME	*Angelica archangelica, Angelica officinalis*
NOTE	top
METHOD OF EXTRACTION	steam distillation
PARTS USED	seeds
FRAGRANCE	fresh, spicy
COLOR(S)	white
CHAKRA(S)	crown, throat, third eye
ASTROLOGICAL SIGN(S)	Aquarius, Pisces
PLANET(S)	Jupiter, Neptune, Uranus
NUMBER(S)	11, 22
ANIMAL(S)	bat, unicorn
ELEMENT(S)	air

Affirmation Guidance and inspiration from my angels and other spirit guides come to me moment by moment. I am a conduit of the Divine. Peace, calm, and serenity are mine, now and always. I am content. I go with the ever-changing flow of life willingly and joyfully.

Complementary flower essences *Aspen* to reassure and relieve anxiousness. *Mimulus* to bring courage and reduce shyness. *Rock Rose* to encourage fearlessness.

Complementary stones Angelite, blue calcite, blue lace agate, celestite, cobaltoan calcite, elestial quartz, channeling quartz, pink tourmaline, smoky quartz, unakite.

About the plant Angelica is a leafy bush with pointed leaves and hollowed ribbed stems that are purple at the bottom and blend into pale green at the top of the stem.

Chemical components Phellandrene, limonene, pinene, caryophyllene.

Spiritual uses Angelica amplifies the ability of the mind and spirit to remember and know the existence of the heavenly messengers who assist you in your daily activities. Use this oil to attract Divine intervention through communication with the angels. Use this oil in synergies or blends to open yourself up to communication with the angelic realm and the realm of invisible helpers. Use it to align with Ascended Masters, especially Saint Germain, and your guardian angels, along with Archangels Auriel, Gabriel, Michael, and Raziel. This oil helps you to focus on astrological or metaphysical pursuits as well as other visionary pursuits. Angelica can also be used to ward off negative energy and release unwanted spirits.

Mental uses Angelica can be used with the intention of calming the mind's incessant chatter. Providing a sense of serenity, this oil is beneficial for times when too many things are happening at once and you need to regain your mental focus. It is a good oil to add to a synergistic blend with the intention of promoting inner peace and restful sleep.

Emotional uses Angelica can help release emotional wounds. It supports release through dreaming, journaling, crying, emoting, and/or processing your emotions. Use this oil to garner support from the angels for help clearing away unnecessary emotional baggage and outside negative influences. Angelica is uplifting and raises your vibration.

Physical uses Angelica improves the ability to sweat, the natural method for removing toxins and waste products from the body. This reduces blood pressure and inhibits fat accumulation in the body. The removal of uric acid and other toxins can offer relief from rheumatism and arthritis. Angelica is helpful for relieving anxiety, nervous exhaustion, bronchitis, asthma, sciatica, headaches, infections, anorexia, anemia, and psoriasis. Angelica is a good aromatherapy ally for intuitive readers, meditation practitioners, mental health counselors, metaphysicians, musicians, mystics, neurologists, and speakers.

Therapeutic properties Analgesic, antibacterial, antifungal, anti-inflammatory, antirheumatic, antiseptic, antispasmodic, antitussive, antiviral, aperitive, aphrodisiac, carminative, cephalic, cicatrizant, depurative, diaphoretic, digestive, diuretic, emmenagogic, estrogenic, febrifugal, hepatic, nervine, revitalizing, stimulative (uterine; nerves), stomachic, sudorific, tonic.

Divine guidance How strong is your connection with your guides and angels? Can you hear the angels? Are you receiving messages from the Divine? Embrace your gift to live a charmed and enlightened life, and to help others attain freedom from suffering and to find happiness and peace. Pursue training to develop your intuitive gifts.

For your safety This oil is phototoxic; therefore, avoid exposure to direct sunlight when using topically. Do not use if pregnant or nursing.

> ### Interesting tidbits:
> Angelica is believed to have made its way from Africa to Europe in the sixteenth century; it was purportedly used to stave off the plague. The stems were chewed to prevent infection. Smudging or burning the seeds and roots disinfects the air. The roots were used in the washing and sanitizing of clothing and linens. Angelica seed is contained in some liquors like Chartreuse, Bénédictine, Vermouth, and Dubonnet.

ANISE SEED
Integration

BOTANICAL NAME	*Pimpinella anisum*
NOTE	top
METHOD OF EXTRACTION	steam distillation
PARTS USED	seeds
FRAGRANCE	sweet, warm, licorice-like aroma; reminiscent of Italian cookies
COLOR(S)	green, orange, yellow
CHAKRA(S)	heart, navel, solar plexus
ASTROLOGICAL SIGN(S)	Aries, Cancer, Leo, Virgo, Scorpio
PLANET(S)	Jupiter, Moon, Neptune, Sun
NUMBER(S)	3
ANIMAL(S)	butterfly, moth, sloth
ELEMENT(S)	air

Affirmation I easily move forward in life, using the lessons of my past as positive stepping stones to my future. My digestive system is healthy. I easily absorb and process all that goes on around me. It is easy for me to stay focused and alert.

Complementary flower essences Holly to release fears of jealousy as well as your own jealousy of others. *Honeysuckle* to observe the past and use the memories to move forward in life. *Larch* to amplify self-confidence and courage. *Walnut* for change and integration. *Willow* to forgive and forget past injustices.

Complementary stones Apatite, citrine, peridot, carnelian, chrysocolla, jade, rose quartz.

About the plant Anise is a herbaceous annual flowering plant with feathery leaves, growing to three feet or more. The flowers are white, producing an aniseed.

Chemical components Anethole, limonene, estragole, anisyl alcohol, himachalene, anisaldehyde, isoeugenyl methyl butyrate.

Spiritual uses Anise seed helps in the prevention of nightmares. Place a few drops on a tissue under your pillow and set the intention to have sweet dreams. Use anise seed in a synergistic blend intended for protection or to increase your intuition and open the third eye chakra.

Mental uses Use anise seed to gain mental clarity and restore attention to a tired mind. This oil promotes active listening skills, bringing the tools of focus and attentiveness into one's qualities. Inhale this essential oil while you repeat the affirmations above.

Emotional uses Use anise seed to assist you when you use the tool of recapitulation for healing and transformative work. Recapitulation helps you remember the belief systems to be released because they no longer serve you. This oil is perfect for women who are preparing for motherhood but are not yet pregnant (see "for your safety" below). Adding a few drops to an aroma-energetic mist is perfect for setting the intention of fertility and making a step toward conscious parenting before conception.

Physical uses Anise seed assists with symptoms of asthma, bronchitis, coughs, flatulence, headaches, indigestion, insect bites, nausea, stomach cramps, and stress. It has an affinity for the digestive system. This oil balances the absorption of sugar and lowers blood sugar levels. While this is a general stimulant for the cardiac, respiratory, and digestive systems, it also acts as a sedative for these systems. It has been used in combination with ylang-ylang to get rid of lice. This oil also makes a good aromatherapy ally for chefs and bakers, as it calls forth the creative spirit of the art of cooking. Anise seed is also a good ally for law enforcement professionals and mothers.

Therapeutic properties Analgesic, antiseptic, antispasmodic, antitussive, aperitive, calmative, carminative, digestive, diuretic, emmenagogic, galactagogic, hypoglycemient, stimulative, stomachic.

Divine guidance Are you unable to integrate what's going on in your life? Are you finding it difficult to *swallow* challenges? The inability to process what is going on around you has a tendency to manifest as indigestion and an upset stomach. Sometimes, when we don't let go of an upsetting thought, feeling, or emotion, it can contribute to constipation.

For your safety Use sparingly or occasionally, as overuse can be carcinogenic. Possible skin irritant. Use with caution if on diabetes medication, as it affects blood sugar levels. Avoid use in cases of endometriosis and estrogen-dependent cancers. Do not use if pregnant or nursing.

Interesting tidbits:
Used medicinally since prehistoric times, anise seed is a staple in aromatherapy. Its use as a food flavoring dates back to the Middle Ages. Anise seed is a member of the parsley family, and its flavor resembles licorice. Egyptians used it in bread, Romans used it as an aphrodisiac, Greeks used it to calm the digestive system, and my Italian grandma used it as a tea for indigestion or a cold. She even used it in her tomato sauce and other traditional dishes.

BASIL
Creative Clarity

BOTANICAL NAME	*Ocimum basilicum*
NOTE	top to middle
METHOD OF EXTRACTION	steam distillation
PARTS USED	leaves and flowering tops
FRAGRANCE	crisp, clean
COLOR(S)	green
CHAKRA(S)	third eye, navel, root
ASTROLOGICAL SIGN(S)	Leo
PLANET(S)	Sun
NUMBER(S)	0, 1, 10
ANIMAL(S)	dolphin, elephant, sloth, white buffalo, white whale
ELEMENT(S)	air

Affirmation I am the ruler of my own kingdom. I express my personal power with grace. I have clarity. If I become distracted, I easily refocus my efforts. I see life from the greater perspective. I am safe and sound.

Complementary flower essences Cerato for decisiveness. *Clematis* for focus. *Mimulus* for courage. *Walnut* to repel challenging people and align with changes. *Wild Oat* to promote decisiveness and action.

Complementary stones Charoite, smoky quartz.

About the plant With over 150 different varieties, basil is a bushy plant that grows to a height of about two feet and has white, blue, or purple flowers.

Chemical components Eugenol, ocimene, isoeugenol, caryophyllene, methyl eugenol, estragole.

Spiritual uses Basil can be used to help you remember spiritual abundance and awaken your connection with protective guides and angels, including Archangel Michael and Sabrael. Use basil as an ingredient in a protection blend to ward off jealousy. It can be used as part of a synergistic blend to help facilitate past-life memories for the purpose of awakening your consciousness in this lifetime. It helps you to call upon Archangel Metatron to bring awareness to your soul's evolutionary process. For a past-life blend, use it with complementary oils, including lemon and rosemary, to heighten mental clarity and memory.

Mental uses Basil aids in mental clarity and memory improvement. This oil helps to shift the way you think about yourself regarding your self-worth and your ability to lead and make great achievements. *Basilicum* comes from the Greek word *Basilicos,* meaning "king" or "royal," so use this oil to recognize the royal within. Employ the law of attraction and use basil to increase your belief in your ability to attract great wealth. Basil untangles chaotic thoughts and sheds light on confusing circumstances and complex situations.

Emotional uses Basil is helpful for gaining an understanding of why you feel the way you do during times of confusing, raging emotions. It relaxes the feeling that others are causing your emotional distress and brings the reins of your emotions back into your own hands to aid in reclaiming emotional control and balance. Basil can help you expand your ability to set boundaries and amplify your personal power. Basil promotes courage and confidence. Basil can help in cases of dementia, according to Valerie Ann Worwood in her book *The Fragrant Mind,* and I found the same to be true as a caregiver for my own father.

Physical uses Use basil to increase your prosperity and entrepreneurial abilities. Because it promotes clear thinking, basil supports your ideas and the know-how to bring them into reality. Use basil to achieve success in business. It is beneficial to deflect negative challenges and helps to maintain focus on following a good plan of action. Basil is a good aromatherapy ally for bankers, brokers, entrepreneurs, finance managers, leaders, law enforcement professionals, marriage counselors, merchants, phlebotomists, and regression therapists.

Therapeutic properties Abortifacient, analgesic, antibacterial, antibiotic, antidepressant, antiparasitic, antiseptic, antispasmodic, antistress, antitussive, antivenomous, aperitive, aphrodisiac, blood purifier, carminative, cephalic, diaphoretic, digestive, emmenagogic, estrogenic, febrifugal, galactagogic, insecticide, laxative, nervine, restorative, sedative, stimulative, stomachic, sudorific, tonic.

Divine guidance Are you feeling like life is out of your control? Are you trying to ward off negative thinking, negative people, and/or negative situations? Know that you are safe and sound. Take time to go within and call upon the royalty within you to reign over your destiny. When you embrace your personal power, you will transform your life.

For your safety Use sparingly or occasionally as it inhibits blood clotting, is potentially carcinogenic, and can be a mild skin and mucous membrane irritant. Avoid use on sensitive skin. Do not use if pregnant or nursing. Do not use with children under age sixteen.

Interesting tidbits:

In some cultures, basil is used as a protective plant for the home, placed by the front and/or back door. This culinary herb is an excellent plant for a kitchen herb garden. Basil is used in many Italian dishes. I use basil as one of the ingredients in a blend to help ward off challenging issues while following a decisive plan to achieve successful ventures. Basil is sacred to the Hindu deities Krishna and Vishnu.

BENZOIN
Stabilize and Transform

Botanical name	*Styrax benzoin*
Note	base
Method of extraction	cold press
Parts used	tree resin
Fragrance	comforting, soft, sweet, vanilla-like
Color(s)	brown, magenta, pink, purple
Chakra(s)	crown, root
Astrological sign(s)	Scorpio, Taurus
Planet(s)	Pluto, Saturn
Number(s)	77, 8
Animal(s)	hawk, owl, raven, snake
Element(s)	fire

Affirmation I unlock the secrets of my soul. My thoughts and belief systems are revealed, clarifying my soul's purpose. It's easy for me to transform negative patterns. I focus my awareness on the unlimited potential available to all.

Complementary flower essences Clematis to focus in on your dreams. *Scleranthus* to activate decisiveness. *Wild Oat* to gain clarity on your soul's purpose.

Complementary stones Amethyst, black tourmaline, brown agate, charoite, hematite, magenta-dyed agate, rose quartz, selenite, smoky quartz.

About the plant Native to Asia, benzoin is a tree that grows up to 115 feet with resinous, aromatic bark and white flowers.

Chemical components Benzyl benzoate, benzyl alcohol, cinnamyl, cinnamate, cinnamic acid, ethyl cinnamate, benzoic acid.

Spiritual uses Benzoin has a strong energetic association with Saint Germain and the Violet Flame. Use it for transformation and alchemical initiations or rites of passage. Add this resin to a synergistic blend to increase the mystical connection beyond conscious awareness. It encourages transformation through dreams and powerful meditation experiences. Benzoin resin adds a magical and mysterious vibration to help you tap into the many levels of awareness. Use this resin to align with your soul contract and to help you do what you came to this planet to do.

Mental uses When used with intention, benzoin can help you gain mental clarity through focused thinking. Begin with a logical approach and then allow the transformative qualities of this resin to guide your thinking to higher knowledge and, ultimately, wisdom. Benzoin helps you seek out answers from elders and experts who have traveled the path you are on.

Emotional uses Benzoin's vanilla-like scent instills a sense of calm, invoking feelings of safety and peace. Include this oil to strengthen the base scent and vibration of protection blends.

Physical uses Benzoin is beneficial for reducing inflammation and muscular tension. It can be used topically in combination with a carrier oil or lotion for skin ulcers, bedsores, and cracked skin. It is a good skin protectant. Use it to improve breathing and various respiratory conditions as it is a mild expectorant. Benzoin also helps to increase circulation. It stabilizes the volatile nature of an essential oil blend. Use it in a synergistic blend to hold the scent and as a grounding agent. Benzoin is a good aromatherapy ally for aromatherapists, body workers, contractors, counselors, ghost hunters, hospice caregivers, law enforcement professionals, librarians, mediators, teachers, and visionary leaders.

Therapeutic properties Anesthetic, antibacterial, antidepressant, anti-inflammatory, antimutagenic, antioxidant, antiparasitic, antipruritic, antiseptic, antispasmodic, antistress, antitussive, antiviral, aphrodisiac, astringent, carminative, cephalic, cicatrizant, cordial, deodorizer, disinfectant, diuretic, drying, euphoriant, fixative, insecticidal, laxative, preservative, rejuvenator, sedative, soothing, stimulative (circulatory system), tonic, uplifting, vulnerary.

Divine guidance Are you heading in too many directions? Do you find that you are spinning in circles and repeating the same challenge again and again? Use this swirling energy to spiral upward and transform your life through higher observation, bringing about positive change. Send out a prayer request for assistance to take the necessary steps to be happy, grounded, and focused, and to live your higher purpose.

For your safety Avoid if taking lithium. Use small amounts and additional carrier oil when applying to the skin because benzoin is more viscous and concentrated than most of the other oils. Do not use if pregnant or nursing.

> ### Interesting tidbits:
> Benzoin is sometimes referred to as Benjamin, which is the name of the tree from which it comes. The resin has been used as incense during religious ceremonies for thousands of years.

BERGAMOT

It's All Good

BOTANICAL NAME	*Citrus bergamia*
NOTE	top to middle
METHOD OF EXTRACTION	cold-press
PARTS USED	fruit peel
FRAGRANCE	fresh, orange-lemony, citrusy, sweet
COLOR(S)	white, green, yellow
CHAKRA(S)	crown, solar plexus
ASTROLOGICAL SIGN(S)	Cancer, Pisces, Leo
PLANET(S)	Moon, Neptune, Pallas Athene, Sun
NUMBER(S)	3
ANIMAL(S)	hummingbird, spider
ELEMENT(S)	air

Affirmation My thoughts amplify my self-confidence and courage. I act fearlessly in the world. I am enthusiastic. I take pleasure in complimenting and encouraging others. Joy is a normal part of my life. My digestive system is healthy. I easily absorb and process all that goes on around me.

Complementary flower essences *Cerato* for guidance and self-confidence. *Elm* to overcome feelings of depression. *Larch* for confidence. *Willow* to think positively.

Complementary stones Amethyst, apatite, citrine, clear quartz, golden calcite, lepidolite, peridot, selenite, yellow jasper.

About the plant Bergamot is an evergreen citrus tree about 15 feet tall that bears yellow-green fragrant fruit the size of an orange.

Chemical components Limonene, linalyl acetate, linalool, sabinene, terpinene, pinene, myrcene, neryl acetate.

Spiritual uses Bergamot helps open pathways in the mind and brain to access higher realms of consciousness as well as information from other realms of existence. Use bergamot during meditation with the intention of aligning your awareness with spiritual master teachers, Ascended Masters, angels, and spirit guides. Bergamot is aligned with Archangels Gabriel and Michael. It activates the essence of Pallas Athene as goddess of wisdom and truth. This oil helps souls remember their connection to the Order of Melchizedek in association with Atlantis and the reactivation of the Grids of Light.

Mental uses The clean, fresh aroma of bergamot is a palate cleanser to the mind. Use it to clear away fogginess and to bring focus and clarity. This uplifting oil aids in thinking good thoughts about yourself and increases your awareness of all your positive qualities.

Emotional uses Bergamot is a good main component in a synergistic blend dedicated to raising your level of joy while releasing any feelings of the blues or symptoms of depression. Inhale this essential oil while you repeat the affirmations above.

Physical uses Bergamot is beneficial physically at the solar plexus chakra in relation to its ability to activate digestive enzymes and bile. Bergamot is a perfect addition to a synergistic blend for the purpose of deodorizing. Add some petitgrain and lemongrass with bergamot to create a natural aromatic and disinfecting mist to clear away pet odors and other unpleasant smells. Use this oil to relax muscles and nerves as well as to relieve cramps. Bergamot is beneficial to improve healing time of wounds because of its antibiotic and antiseptic qualities. Bergamot is a good aromatherapy ally for authors, counselors, dieticians, drug rehabilitation specialists, editors, gastroenterologists, intuitive readers, judges, lawyers, leaders, meditation facilitator/practitioners, mystics, and neurologists.

Therapeutic properties Analgesic, antibiotic, antidepressant, antiparasitic, antiseptic, antispasmodic, antistress, antitoxic, antitussive, aperitive, calmative, carminative, cicatrizant, cordial, deodorizer, digestive, febrifugal, insecticidal, laxative, refreshing, rubefacient, sedative, stomachic, tonic, uplifting, vulnerary.

Divine guidance Are you having a hard time sorting out all the details of what's going on around you and within you? Do you need to gain some understanding to get clear on what direction you want to head? It is time to examine yourself and life through quiet contemplation. Make it your intention to connect with higher spiritual wisdom, and trust that information and knowledge will flow through you.

For your safety This oil is phototoxic (and potentially photocarcinogenic); therefore, avoid exposure to direct sunlight when using topically. Do not use old or oxidized bergamot. Do not use if pregnant or nursing.

> **Interesting tidbits:**
> Bergamot gives the citrusy flavor to Earl Grey tea and Turkish Delight recipes. Bergamot gave the original eighteenth-century German Eau de Cologne its distinct fragrance. I use bergamot in my formulas to raise levels of confidence, happiness, and the ability to embrace life fully and completely.

BIRCH
Ah, Sweet Relief

BOTANICAL NAME	*Betula lenta*
NOTE	top
METHOD OF EXTRACTION	steam distillation
PARTS USED	leaves
FRAGRANCE	clean, deep, medicinal, sharp, sweet, wintergreen, woody
COLOR(S)	white, blue
CHAKRA(S)	third eye
ASTROLOGICAL SIGN(S)	Capricorn, Aquarius, Libra, Gemini
PLANET(S)	Mercury, Saturn, Venus
NUMBER(S)	6
ANIMAL(S)	beaver, peacock
ELEMENT(S)	air

Affirmation I am grateful for the balanced flow of energy within me. My physical structure is strong. All parts of my body feel good. My life is engaging, dynamic, and vibrant. I am full of vigor!

Complementary flower essences Hornbeam to overcome exhaustion. *Oak* for balance of rest and work. *Olive* for rejuvenation.

Complementary stones Azurite, carnelian, chrysocolla, lapis lazuli, orange calcite, rose quartz, sodalite.

About the plant Birch is a deciduous tree reaching heights of up to 50–75 feet tall.

Chemical components Methyl salicylate, ethyl salicylate, linalyl acetate.

Spiritual uses Birch oil is a good addition to diffusion blends for cleansing the aura and releasing toxic energy. While Archangel Raphael is associated with all the essential oils, birch is one that has a stronger association because of its physical pain-relieving properties. On a spiritual level, birch cleans out negative energies accumulated from the past and present, aligning you more fully with your connection to your spiritual path.

Mental uses Birch fosters mental clarity. The vibration of birch increases your ability to act on your dreams and construct your reality. It helps enliven the mind to allow forward movement of the thinking process. Inhale birch when you need mental stimulation. Just as this essential oil flushes toxins out of the physical body, it also cleans out toxic thoughts when used with intention.

Emotional uses Birch energetically assists in reducing inflamed states of consciousness. Breathe deeply to inhale this aroma, which is also the safest way to use this essential oil. This essential oil helps you take in a deep breath of life and overcome painful life challenges. Birch improves your mood and relieves tension.

Physical uses Birch essential oil eases muscle aches, stimulates circulation, and reduces swelling. It helps relieve arthritis pain and reduces inflammation. It eliminates the accumulation of uric acid in the joints. It helps to flush out the kidneys and increases the flow of urine. It is helpful to relieve eczema, psoriasis, and acne. Birch reduces fevers and encourages perspiration, which also helps to clear toxins. Birch is a good aromatherapy ally for athletes, body workers, caregivers, dental professionals, healthcare practitioners, hospice caregivers, marathon participants, nurses, physical therapists, physical trainers, Reiki practitioners, shamanic practitioners, and spiritual healers.

Therapeutic properties Analgesic, anti-inflammatory, antiparasitic, antirheumatic, antiseptic, antitoxic, astringent, depurative, detersive, disinfectant, diuretic, febrifugal, insecticidal, laxative, rubefacient, stimulative (circulatory system), tonic.

Divine guidance Are you ready to take action to achieve your dreams and desires? Do you believe you are able to overcome the challenges? It's time to move beyond the pains of your past and build the joys of your future. Breathe deeply and take action to move forward with ease and grace to create your reality.

For your safety Avoid if allergic to aspirin, if on anticoagulants, and in cases of high blood pressure. Do not use if pregnant or nursing. Do not use on children under age 19.

> **Interesting tidbits:**
> The fragrance of sweet birch exudes directly from the bark of the birch tree. Native Americans use birch leaves and dried bark in purification ceremonies, such as sweat lodges.

CARDAMOM
Digest Life

BOTANICAL NAME	*Elettaria cardamomum*
NOTE	middle
METHOD OF EXTRACTION	steam distillation
PARTS USED	seeds prior to ripening
FRAGRANCE	spicy, sweet, pungent, warm
COLOR(S)	clear, pale yellow
CHAKRA(S)	crown, solar plexus
ASTROLOGICAL SIGN(S)	Cancer, Virgo
PLANET(S)	Moon
NUMBER(S)	9
ANIMAL(S)	hawk, vulture
ELEMENT(S)	fire

Affirmation I easily accept whatever happens in my life. I readily absorb and process my experiences and all that goes on around me. My digestive system is healthy. I am able to discern the truth and take positive action by using the wisdom of the elders and ancestors. I am a channel of love, light, and well-being.

Complementary flower essences Hornbeam for feeling overwhelmed. *Mimulus* for integration, oversensitivity, and worry over the future. *Mustard* to raise you from being depressed.

Complementary stones Apatite, citrine, channeling quartz, fluorite, golden calcite, peridot, trilobite fossil.

About the plant Cardamom is a perennial bush in the ginger family that grows to about 10 feet.

Chemical components Cineole, terpinyl acetate, linalyl acetate, limonene, linalool, terpineol, sabinene, terpinen, nerolidol, myrcene, pinene, geraniol.

Spiritual uses Cardamom helps to optimize your personal filtering system when you are receiving channeled messages from the ancestors on the Other Side. In highly sensitive and intuitive individuals, it aids in activating and maintaining a clear crown chakra to receive the wisdom of the ages. It also helps to keep unwelcome energies from interfering with the channeling process so that you can be a pure channel.

Mental uses Cardamom alleviates mental fatigue and improves the thought processes. This spicy oil offers mental clarity. Cardamom is useful when you need support dealing with the minutiae of your life. With its ability to help you sort through what's important and what isn't, it is especially beneficial for anyone who works in any capacity with details and scheduling or organization.

Emotional uses Add cardamom to a synergistic blend to help move you out of depressed states and boost your spirits. Cardamom aligns you with the ability to integrate all that is happening around you. This digestive oil assists you in digesting life and in gaining the realization that you only need to retain what nourishes you emotionally and mentally, and then release what no longer serves your highest good. Cardamom helps you determine which feelings are yours and which feelings have been imposed upon you by society or other people.

Physical uses The vibration of cardamom helps you decide on a plan for healthy eating. In *The Fragrant Mind*, Worwood indicates that cardamom is an appetite stimulant and memory-evoking oil helpful in cases of dementia and Alzheimer's disease. Cardamom is beneficial to calm intestinal spasms and flatulence and to clear away parasites. Use cardamom to balance the gallbladder and the liver, as well as your appetite. Because it is a diuretic, cardamom also lowers blood pressure. In its role as an anti-inflammatory, it's useful to combat colds, flus, and bronchial challenges. Cardamom is a good aromatherapy ally for counselors, dieticians, engineers, gastroenterologists, intuitive readers, judges, and musicians.

Therapeutic properties Antimicrobial, antiparasitic, antiseptic, antispasmodic, aphrodisiac, antitussive, carminative, cephalic, digestive, diuretic, stimulative, stomachic, tonic.

Divine guidance Do you often feel inspired? Are you a channel who receives messages from angels and loved ones on the Other Side? Take the time to clear your consciousness to discern the truth. Make it your intention to gain clarity in your life. Ask your ancestors, spirit guides, and angels for understanding or clarity; then be ready to receive the inspiration.

For your safety Do not use if pregnant or nursing. Keep away from the face of infants and children.

> **Interesting tidbits:**
> Ancient Egyptians chewed cardamom seeds for dental hygiene. It was used in the Middle East as an aphrodisiac.

CEDARWOOD
Protect and Cleanse

BOTANICAL NAME	*Juniperus virginiana*
NOTE	base
METHOD OF EXTRACTION	steam distillation
PARTS USED	bark, sawdust, wood, and wood chips
FRAGRANCE	earthy, woody; reminiscent of the forest
COLOR(S)	green, yellow
CHAKRA(S)	root, solar plexus, heart
ASTROLOGICAL SIGN(S)	Capricorn
PLANET(S)	Earth, Saturn
NUMBER(S)	69/6
ANIMAL(S)	beetle, dragonfly, white buffalo
ELEMENT(S)	earth

Affirmation With every step I take, I am aware of my connection with the sacred ground. The vibrant emerald-green energy of the plants and trees nurtures and restores my body, mind, and spirit. Everything I need to know is stored within me. I easily tap into my inner wisdom and knowledge.

Complementary flower essences Clematis for focus. *Red Chestnut* for peace of mind. *Walnut* for protection.

Complementary stones Blue lace agate, citrine, green moss agate, hematite, petrified wood, tree agate.

About the plant Virginian cedarwood is an evergreen tree that grows to a height of over 100 feet. Part of the genus *Juniper*, it is not a true cedar.

Chemical components Cedrene, thujopsene, cedrol, selinene, widdrol, himachalene, chamigrene, cuparene.

Spiritual uses Add cedarwood to synergistic blends intended to clear away negativity. Just as sage and cedar are traditionally burned together for ceremonial use and smudging, use the essential oils of sage and cedarwood together in an aroma-energetic mist to spritz away negative energy. Cedarwood is helpful for meditation and prayer work. Cedarwood deepens your spiritual practice and rituals. It is useful when you want to ground a visualization practice or focused intent to draw upon the gifts of the law of attraction. It helps bring about prophetic visions.

Mental uses Use cedarwood oil to help you remember to ground yourself. Use it when you are experiencing mental fatigue in order to replenish your mental focus. Cedarwood has a grounding effect and aids those challenged by the symptoms of attention deficit hyperactivity disorder (ADHD). The energy of the tree helps you to strengthen your inner potentials.

Emotional uses Cedarwood helps you reclaim your balance through nature. Allow this oil to encourage you to spend time outdoors to release emotional challenges. While in nature, use this oil to imagine emotional toxins draining from the soles of your feet into the ground. Cedarwood oil can be used to calm your nerves, helping to reduce stress and anxiety.

Physical uses Cedarwood has been used to reduce blood pressure. It is helpful for many skin conditions, including cracked skin, eczema, psoriasis, and acne. Cedarwood can be used as an aid to prevent baldness. Use cedarwood in synergistic blends to relieve congestion and open breathing passages. Cedarwood repels moths. This oil is used to reduce muscle aches and the symptoms of rheumatism and arthritis. Cedar trees have the vibration of Earth Keeper, a steward of this planet. Cedarwood is a good aromatherapy ally for arborists, dermatologists, ecologists, environmentalists, ghost hunters, housekeepers, infectious disease specialists, landscape architects, law enforcement professionals, meditation facilitators/practitioners, neurologists, and shamanic practitioners.

Therapeutic properties Antipruritic, antiseptic, antispasmodic, astringent, antiseborrheic, antitussive, balsamic, diuretic, emmenagogic, emollient, insecticidal, healing (skin), sedative.

Divine guidance Do you want to amplify your focus and ability to ground your spiritual experiences? Allow the qualities of cedarwood to amplify your focus and the preservation of knowledge, wisdom, love, and protection. Have you been spending time in nature? Whether you live in a small city apartment or on an expansive farm, you can always find a way to establish your roots into the earth and nature. Use the negative ions of the mountains, sea, or air, which provide positive energy for bringing about balance for your overall good.

For your safety Do not use if pregnant or nursing.

> **Interesting tidbits:**
> Traditionally used in Native American Indian ceremonies for prayer and blessings, cedarwood is often included in smudging blends to replace negativity with positive energy. Ancient Egyptians used cedarwood oil in the embalming process. Cedar boughs have been used to decorate Yule logs.

CELERY SEED

Let go

BOTANICAL NAME	*Apium graveolens*
NOTE	middle to base
METHOD OF EXTRACTION	steam distillation
PARTS USED	seeds
FRAGRANCE	celery-like, earthy, fresh, slightly spicy, warm
COLOR(S)	green, olive green, orange, yellow
CHAKRA(S)	navel, solar plexus
ASTROLOGICAL SIGN(S)	Aries, Cancer, Capricorn
PLANET(S)	Mars, Pluto, Saturn
NUMBER(S)	22
ANIMAL(S)	crab, sloth, snake
ELEMENT(S)	air, water

Affirmation I am happy for the good fortune and blessings of others. It is easy for me to stay calm. I let go of what is no longer for my highest good and go with the flow. All my joints are healthy and comfortable. I release anger in a healthy and balanced way. All toxins are easily processed and removed from my body. Events from my past positively affect my present and future.

Complementary flower essences *Holly* to realign feelings of anger, bitterness, and jealousy. *Oak* to help you recover and renew after periods of struggle. *White Chestnut* to release incessant chatter and repetitive thoughts. *Willow* to release self-pity, resentment, and bitterness.

Complementary stones Ametrine, bloodstone, citrine, carnelian, chrysocolla, copper, malachite, peridot, yellow chrysoprase.

About the plant Celery is a biennial plant that grows to a height of 1 to 2 feet with green and white flowers that produce seeds.

Chemical components Limonene, selinene, butylidenephthalide, ligustilide, sedanenolide, pentylbenzene, linalool, myrcene, pinene.

Spiritual uses Use celery seed oil with the intention to increase your ability to tap into the cosmos to garner wisdom, knowledge, and surprising information that can be applied to your spiritual practice of meditation, prayer, and contemplation. Add celery seed oil to a synergistic blend to invoke Archangel Camael with the intention of realigning yourself with love and acceptance (the opposite of anger and aggression).

Mental uses Celery seed oil is energetically beneficial when working on an invention, formula, or any project that requires a download of insight to complete a task at hand. It is beneficial for writers, musicians, and inventors who feel stumped or stagnant. Celery seed oil is beneficial when you can't think clearly because of hurt feelings that cause you to be more suspicious or jealous. Call on Archangel Sabrael to help release feelings of jealousy. Use it with the intention to feel inner peace and release thoughtforms that eventually will only harm you.

Emotional uses Celery seed oil can be added to a synergetic blend for overcoming insecurities and jealousy of others or when you need to have the courage to set boundaries with others. It can help you if you feel hurt by a friend's betrayal or a relationship breakup. It helps to transform and transmute negative emotions and releases the hooks that others may have in your emotional body.

Physical uses Celery seed is best used as a means of ridding your body of excess water through urination. (As a reminder, use this oil in a carrier oil and apply it to the soles of your feet. Do not take this or any other essential oil internally.) It is beneficial to lowering blood pressure. Celery seed oil has components to help cleanse the liver, spleen, and bladder. It increases the elimination of uric acid, which relieves symptoms of gout and neuralgia. It is known to relieve the symptoms of rheumatoid arthritis. Celery seed promotes sleep. Celery seed is a good aromatherapy ally for weight loss counselors and gastroenterologists.

Therapeutic properties Abortifacient, analgesic, antiarthritic, anticonvulsive, antilithic, antioxidant, antiphlogistic, antirheumatic, antiscorbutic, antispasmodic, aperitive, aphrodisiac, carminative, cholagogic, depurative, diaphoretic, digestive, diuretic, emmenagogic, hepatic, hypotensor, nervine, sedative, stimulative (uterine contractions), stomachic, tonic, vulnerary.

Divine guidance Are you receiving a clear signal and comprehensible messages from others and the Universe? Do you feel stagnated? Do you have repetitive thoughts about hurts of the past? It's time to clear your channel. Allow wisdom to flow through you and release what is no longer for your highest good. Believe in yourself. Have confidence in your ability to tap into universal knowledge and wisdom.

For your safety None known.

Interesting tidbits:
In ancient times, Ayurvedic medicine prescribed celery seed for colds, flu, edema, digestion, arthritis, and other ailments.

CHAMOMILE
Go with the Flow

BOTANICAL NAME	*Matricaria chamomilla, Matricaria recutita* (German chamomile), *Anthemis Nobilis* (Roman chamomile)
NOTE	middle
METHOD OF EXTRACTION	steam distillation
PARTS USED	flowers
FRAGRANCE	fruity, herbaceous, distinctive apple-like scent, strong
COLOR(S)	dark navy blue, pastel blue (German); yellow, white, green (Roman)
CHAKRA(S)	third eye, throat (German); solar plexus, heart (Roman)
ASTROLOGICAL SIGN(S)	Pisces, Taurus, Virgo
PLANET(S)	Chiron, Neptune, Sun, Venus
NUMBER(S)	7, 11, 22, 33
ANIMAL(S)	domestic cat, eagle, lizard
ELEMENT(S)	water

Affirmation I am calm. I am at peace. I am content. I go with the ever-changing flow of life willingly and joyfully. I breathe deeply and oxygen replenishes my body. I feel protected.

Complementary flower essences Aspen for reassurance. *Cherry Plum* for composure. *Impatiens* for patience. *Star of Bethlehem* for comfort. *White Chestnut* for inner peace.

Complementary stones Angelite, apatite, azurite, celestite, dyed blue agate, lapis lazuli, sodalite (German), citrine, goldstone, green moss agate, sunstone, tree agate (Roman).

About the plant Chamomile, often found growing wild, has small flowers with white petals and yellow centers, reminiscent of tiny daisies. German chamomile grows up to 3 feet tall and Roman chamomile grows to about a foot tall.

Chemical components Bisabolol oxide, farnesene, chamazulene, spiroethers, bisabolol (German), isobutyl angelate, butyl angelate, methylpentyl angelate, isotuyl butyrate, isoamyl angelate, methyl propenyl angelate, methylpentyl isobutyrate, methyl propyl angelate, camphene, borneol, pinene, terpinene, chamazulene, pinocarveol, thujene, hexyl butyrate, anthemol, isoamyl isobutyrate, carene, isoamyl methylbutyrate, methylbutyl methylbutyrate, isoamyl butyrate, pinocarvone, myrcene, cymene, isoamyl methacrylate, phellandrene, propyl angelate (Roman).

Spiritual uses German chamomile assists with spiritual connection to guides and angels through dreamtime. Place a drop on a tissue or cotton ball and inhale prior to meditation or sleep (being mindful that the blue azulene can stain). German chamomile is good for connecting with Archangel Michael. Roman chamomile is helpful to connect with Archangel Gabriel for introspection and reflection. Roman chamomile's golden vibration is beneficial to align with Archangel Uriel to activate your connection with creativity, universal flow, and inner peace.

Mental uses Use German and Roman chamomile to calm the incessant chatter in your mind. This oil relieves stress by helping to heal frayed nerves. Its calming effects help you sort out your thoughts. This is a good oil to use to cancel out angry, vindictive, or negative thoughts.

Emotional uses Intense emotions and outbursts can be allayed through the use of this oil. Allow the blue energy to release negative emotions and calm you. Inhaling German chamomile lets you know that all is well. German and Roman chamomile help to quell emotional outbursts brought on by premenstrual syndrome (PMS), menopause, or any other hormone-related upsets. They also calm insomnia. Use Roman chamomile to improve self-esteem and reduce anxiety.

Physical uses This essential oil can be used to relieve inflamed joints and is effective in the treatment of sprains and inflammations of all kinds. Azulene—the blue component in German chamomile—relieves indigestion, acid reflux, boils, and acne. Both German and Roman chamomile promote restful sleep. Chamomile is beneficial in releasing physical symptoms of PMS and menstrual pain. German and Roman chamomile also help to reduce fevers. German chamomile is a good aromatherapy ally for athletes, clairvoyants, intuitive readers, meditation facilitators/practitioners, physical therapists, physical trainers, and teachers. Roman chamomile is a good aromatherapy ally for gastroenterologists, inventors, meditation facilitators/practitioners, neurologists, shamanic practitioners, and speakers.

Therapeutic properties Analgesic, antianemic, antibacterial, antibiotic, anticonvulsive, antidepressant, antifungal, anti-inflammatory, antineuralgic, antiparasitic, antipruritic, antirheumatic, antiseptic, antispasmodic, antitoxic, aperitive, calmative, carminative, cholagogic, cicatrizant, diaphoretic, digestive, diuretic, emmenagogic, emollient, hepatic, hypotensor, laxative, nervine, sedative, stomachic, sudorific, tonic, vulnerary.

Divine guidance Have you been experiencing physical inflammation or hormone imbalances? Is a situation in your life inflamed? Steps to reduce emotional, physical, and mental inflammation are in order. Try visualization and meditation with this essential oil to bring a new calmness to every aspect of yourself. Peace and tranquility are yours for the asking.

For your safety Avoid if allergic to asters, daisies, chrysanthemums, or ragweed. Do not use if pregnant or nursing. Roman chamomile should be avoided in the first trimester of pregnancy.

> ### *Interesting tidbits:*
> The azulene content in the German chamomile gives it a deep blue color, which can stain clothing and linens.

Cinnamon
The Spice of Life

Botanical name	*Cinnamomum zeylanicum*
Note	middle to base
Method of extraction	steam distillation
Parts used	leaves
Fragrance	musky, sharp, spicy, strong, sweet
Color(s)	beige, brown, orange
Chakra(s)	navel, solar plexus, third eye
Astrological sign(s)	Leo, Sagittarius
Planet(s)	Jupiter, Mercury, Sun, Venus
Number(s)	9
Animal(s)	elephant, goldfish, owl, raven
Element(s)	fire

Affirmation Abundance and prosperity are constantly flowing in my life. I am courageous. I bravely bring my ideas into actuality. My imagination is the key to my success. My ideas are fresh and creative. I take action to manifest my artistic thoughts. I embrace life and enjoy a strong passion for living.

Complementary flower essences Gentian to restore hope and confidence to bring ideas to fruition. *Wild Oat* to remove perceived blocks. *Wild Rose* to help to get your creative juices flowing and increase enthusiasm.

Complementary stones Brucite, carnelian, honey calcite, orange calcite, red jasper, smoky quartz, sunstone.

About the plant Cinnamon is an evergreen tree with leathery green leaves; it is often cultivated as a bush.

Chemical components Eugenol, eugenyl acetate, linalool, cinnamyl acetate, benzyl benzoate, caryophyllene, cinnamaldehyde, safrole, cinnamyl alcohol.

Spiritual uses Cinnamon increases psychic awareness. Use this essential oil with the intention of increasing your connection with the Divine and to maximize your intuitive skills, including all the sensory gifts of clairvoyance, clairaudience, claircognizance, clairsentience, clairolfaction, and clairgustation.

Mental uses Use cinnamon to wake you up from a mental stupor, as it boosts cognitive function. It revitalizes blood flow, and as the energy moves, it increases your mental capacity to listen, learn, absorb, and integrate all that is going on around you and within your mind. Cinnamon is beneficial for venturing outside the norm of your regular way of thinking, allowing you to use your mind in different ways to achieve new results in your life.

Emotional uses Cinnamon raises your confidence and self-esteem. It helps to unblock the energy you call "blocks," allowing you to move beyond the perception that something is standing in the way of your goals, desires, or the completion of creative projects. Inhale this essential oil while you repeat the affirmations above. It warms up emotional voids that feel cold and stagnant.

Physical uses Use cinnamon's aroma to increase your appetite. Cinnamon has a warming action that raises the body temperature, which is beneficial for colds and flu relief. It also reduces blood sugar levels, kills fungi and bacteria, increases circulation, and strengthens the heart. Cinnamon also reduces the levels of bad cholesterol and reduces arthritis pain. It has been shown in studies to slow the proliferation of leukemia and lymphoma cancer cells, as well as to reduce or eliminate candida due to its antifungal properties. Cinnamon is a good aromatherapy ally for artists, bakers, entrepreneurs, leaders, merchants, musicians, and inventors.

Therapeutic properties Analgesic, anesthetic, antibacterial, antibiotic, anticonvulsive, antidepressant, antidiabetic, antidiarrheal, antidotal, antiemetic, anti-inflammatory, antioxidant, antiputrid, antiparasitic, antirheumatic, antiseptic (strong), antispasmodic, antitussive, antiviral, aperitive, aphrodisiac, astringent (mild), cardiac, carminative, digestive, emmenagogic, emollient, estrogenic, febrifugal, hemostatic, hepatic, hypoglycemient, insecticidal, stimulative, stomachic, tonic.

Divine guidance Have you wanted to do something creative? Are you feeling artistic? Have you observed that you have a negative attitude that stops you from taking action to complete something? Let your inspiration flow and generate your insight into manifest reality. This is a time of prosperity and purpose. You are ready to step into your power and be all that you were meant to be. You are aligned with the magnificence and the courage to show yourself in your fullest splendor!

For your safety May inhibit blood clotting, so avoid use if on anticoagulants. Do not add to baths as it can be irritating to mucous membranes. Do not use if pregnant or nursing.

Interesting tidbits:

Written records of cinnamon as a spice go back as far as 2700 BC. It is often used as an air freshener in restaurant restrooms to freshen up the air and activate hunger. It is one of the flavoring ingredients in Coca-Cola. The scent of cinnamon attracts prosperity and abundance. I've placed cinnamon sticks beside the cash register at my store for years.

CLARY SAGE
Euphoria

BOTANICAL NAME	*Salvia sclarea*
NOTE	top to middle
METHOD OF EXTRACTION	steam distillation
PARTS USED	flowers and leaves
FRAGRANCE	balsamic, heavy, herbal, nutty, strong, sweet top note, tobacco-like middle note
COLOR(S)	blue, cobalt, yellow
CHAKRA(S)	navel, solar plexus, third eye
ASTROLOGICAL SIGN(S)	Cancer, Pisces
PLANET(S)	Moon, Neptune
NUMBER(S)	1
ANIMAL(S)	horse, hummingbird
ELEMENT(S)	air, water

Affirmation I embrace my emotions as I allow balance to return to my life. Nurturing energy surrounds me. I attract inner peace and great joy every day in many ways. I have the courage to step forward with joy and enthusiasm.

Complementary flower essences Oak to help relax the over-achiever. *Vervain* to temper high tension and hyperactivity. *Vine* to calm aggressiveness. *Walnut* for difficulties during times of change.

Complementary stones Azurite, chrysocolla, citrine, golden calcite, golden topaz, lapis lazuli, lepidolite, pyrite, rose quartz, sodalite, sugilite.

About the plant Native to Europe, clary sage is a potently aromatic plant that grows to a height of about 3 feet. It has blue, pink, or white flowers.

Chemical components Linalyl acetate, linalool, germacrene, sclareol, caryophyllene, copaene, bicyclogermacrene.

Spiritual uses Clary sage is a good essential oil to use for contemplation, meditation, and prayer. Use this essential oil to help release incessant chatter to achieve a deep state of meditation. Clary sage helps you to remain calm when receiving intuitive guidance, allowing you to relax enough to observe and interpret how it applies to your life. Inhale clary sage and call on Archangel Auriel to help release subconscious fears. Call on Archangel Camael to release anger, aggression, and rampant emotions. Clary sage helps to cultivate tools to love and be loved without neediness. Use this oil to develop a true understanding of detachment. It can help you develop healthy relationships through the realization of the impermanent nature of reality.

Mental uses Clary sage relaxes the judgments in the mind, allowing you to let go and let others live their lives. As you release judgment of others and yourself, you become the objective observer.

Emotional uses Clary sage relaxes, comforts, and grounds feelings and emotions. It replaces the energy of hysteria with a sense of well-being and euphoria. It is especially beneficial when emotions are rampant. Use it for calming and releasing anger and frustration. It helps to quell emotional outbursts brought on by premenstrual syndrome, menopause, and other hormone-related upsets. This oil helps you acknowledge and accept hormone-related *realizations* as accurate but also helps you find a way to deal with and express them in a way that other people can handle.

Physical uses Clary sage helps to rebalance overall physical health by helping to release stress and anxiety. Use clary sage to restore strength after an illness. This oil reduces blood pressure, headaches, and migraines through the release of tension. It reduces perspiration. Clary sage is great for sound sleep. Clary sage is an aromatherapy ally for doulas, drug rehabilitation specialists, fertility specialists, gynecologists, hospice caregivers, marriage counselors, meditation facilitators/practitioners, mental health counselors, and sex therapists.

Therapeutic properties Analgesic, anticonvulsive, antidepressant, anti-inflammatory, antiseptic, antispasmodic, antistress, antisudorific, antiviral, aphrodisiac, astringent, balsamic, calmative, carminative, deodorizer, digestive, emmenagogic, emollient, estrogenic, euphoriant, fixative, healing (skin), hypotensor, nervine, refreshing, relaxant (strong), regenerative (skin cells), sedative, stimulant (uterine contractions), stomachic, tonic, tonifying, uplifting, warming.

Divine guidance Is a situation in your life inflamed? Do you grab onto a thought, memory, or life experience and chew it over and over and over again? It is time to let go and release situations from your past—whether it was five minutes ago or five years ago—and find inner peace and true happiness. Steps to reduce emotional, physical, and mental inflammation are in order. Try visualization and meditation to bring a new calmness to every aspect of your life and body.

For your safety Has a sedative effect; avoid prior to driving and when it is necessary to stay alert. Avoid when drinking alcohol, as nausea may result. Avoid in cases of low blood pressure. Use sparingly or occasionally, as overuse may cause headaches. Do not use if pregnant or nursing.

> **Interesting tidbits:**
> In folklore, clary sage is called "clear eye." I use clary sage as an essential ingredient in my blends for relaxation and fertility.

CLOVE
Strength

BOTANICAL NAME	*Eugenia caryophyllata*
NOTE	base
METHOD OF EXTRACTION	steam distillation
PARTS USED	leaves
FRAGRANCE	fruity, spicy, strong, warm
COLOR(S)	brown, orange, white, yellow
CHAKRA(S)	crown, navel, solar plexus, third eye
ASTROLOGICAL SIGN(S)	Aries, Gemini, Sagittarius
PLANET(S)	Jupiter, Mars, Mercury
NUMBER(S)	13, 15/6
ANIMAL(S)	hawk, turtle
ELEMENT(S)	air, fire

Affirmation I am strong. My inner core is powerful. I have the courage to set boundaries with love and grace. I am protected from negative energy. Experiences from the past empower me. Creativity flows through me in myriad ways. I am courageous. I bring my ideas into actuality.

Complementary flower essences Centaury to help you set boundaries and stand up for yourself. *Oak* for feeling weak and worn out. *Olive* to accept rest and to reconnect with life's pleasures.

Complementary stones Amber, aragonite, carnelian, citrine, dogtooth calcite, mookaite jasper, golden calcite, golden topaz, orange calcite, variegated jasper.

About the plant Clove is a tropical flowering evergreen tree that grows to a height of about 40 feet. It has bright pink buds that form into purple berries.

Chemical components Eugenol, caryophyllene, eugenyl acetate, isoeugenol.

Spiritual uses Clove oil is beneficial for protection from ill wishes and negative energy from your own thought patterns. It helps deflect jealousy. Add it to a protective synergistic blend to strengthen internal faith and help you remember that you are divinely protected. The aroma of clove oil can be an ally during regression therapy to help remember and know what is important at this moment for your spiritual evolution. Clove oil partners well with creative visualization techniques to improve all areas of your life.

Mental uses Clove has an uplifting effect on the mind, as its warm energy is mentally stimulating, improving your ability to think clearly, capture ideas, and establish clear steps for bringing ideas to fruition. Inhale the scent of clove oil to improve memory and gain clarity on how to set healthy boundaries with ease and grace.

Emotional uses The spicy vibes of clove fortify the emotional field by raising your energy. It relieves the blues and the symptoms of depression. The vibration of clove strengthens self-confidence. It relieves energetic lethargy and improves your ability to embrace feelings and move forward. To increase courage, sniff clove oil and imagine a positive outcome for the circumstance that requires strength.

Physical uses This is beneficial to disinfect the atmosphere of infectious disease. It is known to relieve flatulence. It has been used for many years to relieve toothaches. Its pain-relieving qualities extend to muscle aches, and in this case, it is especially beneficial in a synergistic blend with birch, wintergreen, and other analgesic oils. Clove is useful for ridding the body of parasites. Clove is a good aromatherapy ally for bakers, body workers, dentists, ear/nose/throat specialists, environmentalists, Feng Shui practitioners, graphic designers, law enforcement professionals, pest control professionals, physical trainers, Pilates instructors, and regression therapists.

Therapeutic properties Abortifacient, analgesic, anesthetic (local), antibacterial, antibiotic, antidepressant, antiemetic, antifungal, antineuralgic, anti-inflammatory, antioxidant, antirheumatic, antiseptic (strong), antispasmodic, antistress, antiparasitic, antitussive, antiviral, aperitive, aphrodisiac, carminative, caustic, cicatrizant, dermatological, emmenagogic, insecticidal, stimulative (vitality), stomachic, tonic.

Divine guidance Are you involved in a creative project or thinking about starting one? Have you been procrastinating lately or avoiding some tasks? You can access good ideas and have the ability to conceive something magnificent. Have the courage to take action to make your dreams and ideas into a reality. Perhaps you've avoided looking at an emotional issue. Take the time to find the root cause of emotional patterns. Remove challenges that have been entrenched in your emotional body and heal once and for all.

For your safety Possible skin irritant. May inhibit blood clotting, so avoid use if on anticoagulants. Do not use with children under age nineteen. Do not use if pregnant or nursing. Clove is one of the ingredients in the original Auntie M's Anti-Disinfecting Oil because of its antibacterial, antifungal, antiseptic, antiviral, and antiparasitic qualities.

> *Interesting tidbits:*
> The earliest known use of clove (circa 220 BC) was by the Chinese, who chewed it to sweeten the breath. It is a traditional ingredient in the United Kingdom in recipes for pies, ham, and marinades. It is used in perfumes like Dana's *Tabu* and Lauder's *Cinnabar*, Laurent's *Opium*, and Chanel's *Coco*.

CORIANDER
Cleansing

BOTANICAL NAME	*Coriandrum sativum*
NOTE	top to middle
METHOD OF EXTRACTION	steam distillation
PARTS USED	seeds
FRAGRANCE	citrusy, earthy, fresh, green, spicy, sweet, woody
COLOR(S)	green, olive, orange, teal, yellow
CHAKRA(S)	navel, solar plexus
ASTROLOGICAL SIGN(S)	Cancer, Capricorn, Virgo
PLANET(S)	Ceres, Mercury, Moon, Saturn
NUMBER(S)	2
ANIMAL(S)	dolphin, frog
ELEMENT(S)	air, water

Affirmation Blessings flow through me like a healing river. I am fluid. I am pure and clear. I take time to relax in a pool, bath, or body of water. I drink the right amount of water to maintain a fluid, healthy body.

Complementary flower essences Chestnut Bud to recognize life patterns and use the lessons learned. *Crab Apple* to feel clean and healthy. *Gentian* for motivation.

Complementary stones Apatite, carnelian, citrine, chlorite phantom quartz, clear quartz, copper, dogtooth calcite, fluorite, golden calcite, green moss agate, Herkimer diamond, howlite, malachite, serpentine, tree agate, unakite, zebra jasper.

About the plant Coriander is a parsley-like plant that reaches a height of about 3 feet. It has white flowers that form into green seeds.

Chemical components Linalool, pinene, terpinene, camphor, geraniol, limonene, geranyl acetate, terpinen, terpineol.

Spiritual uses Just as you may use coriander to flush physical toxins out of your body, you can also use it to cleanse your aura, or energy field. The spiritual wisdom of the plant kingdom and the devic forces of the plants can be accessed by working with this refreshing aroma. This oil opens a doorway to the world of fairies, gnomes, and elves, giving you the opportunity to meet and greet them.

Mental uses Coriander improves memory and mental clarity. This energizing essential oil helps with the physical endurance you need to stay focused on what needs to get done while maintaining the motivation to do it. It helps you concentrate on what you need to do in the moment, rather than on every other thing you need to get done later.

Emotional uses Coriander oil helps when you've decided to rid yourself of emotional baggage that is clogging up your emotional body and preventing healthy relationships. It helps you uncover and release emotions that have been bubbling beneath the surface so that you can proceed toward emotional healing and discontinue unwanted repetitive patterns in your relationships. Use coriander with the intention to take action and move forward in life. It is useful when you are up against an emotional block.

Physical uses The cleansing and refreshing vibration of coriander supports the digestive system. It balances the digestive process and promotes healthy bowel movements. Coriander oil is useful to relieve pain and symptoms of osteoarthritis and rheumatism. It helps to remove the toxins that cause joint pain. Coriander is also a sleep aid. Coriander is a good aromatherapy ally for arborists, aromatherapists, cardiologists, heart surgeons, gardeners, and marriage counselors.

Therapeutic properties Abortifacient, analgesic, anesthetic, antibacterial, anti-inflammatory, antimutagenic, antioxidant, febrifugal, antirheumatic, antispasmodic, antitumor, aperitive, aphrodisiac, calmative, cardiotonic, carminative, deodorizer, depurative, detoxifier, diaphoretic, digestive, diuretic, emmenagogic, hepatic, nervine, refreshing, regenerator, revitalizing, stimulative (circulatory system), stomachic, tonic, uplifting, warming.

Divine guidance Have you been compartmentalizing your feelings and thoughts? It is time to delve into your consciousness through meditation or contemplation to heal old wounds on all levels and venture out into the world once again. Take the time to look at what needs to be cleared away and renewed in your life. Maintain fluidity at all levels of consciousness. Allow the natural flow to detoxify your body, mind, and emotions.

For your safety No known contraindications.

Interesting tidbits:
The herb coriander has been used as a culinary herb and for medicinal purposes since ancient times (dating back to 5000 BC) in Babylon, Egypt, Greece, and Rome. *Cilantro* is the Spanish name for coriander leaves. It is said that the ancient Chinese believed the seeds contained the power of immortality. Coriander is one of the bitter herbs often included in the Passover ritual.

Cypress, Blue
The Underworld and Transformation

Botanical name	*Callitris intratropica*
Note	base to middle
Method of extraction	steam distillation
Parts used	wood
Fragrance	balsamic, fruity, lemony, licorice-like, resinous, smoky, sweet, woody
Color(s)	brown, green, pink, purple
Chakra(s)	navel, root, solar plexus
Astrological sign(s)	Scorpio
Planet(s)	Ceres, Chiron, Pluto
Number(s)	8
Animal(s)	bear, lizard
Element(s)	air

Affirmation I completely embrace the depth of my feelings. I know that any intense feelings of anger, sorrow, and grief will pass as I willingly release them from my body. I connect with loved ones on the Other Side and easily interpret their messages.

Complementary flower essences Mimulus for worry and fear of things known and unknown. *Red Chestnut* for overconcern for the welfare of a deceased loved one. *Walnut* for changes from one way of being to another. *White Chestnut* to calm the mind.

Complementary stones Apache tears, cobra jasper, Herkimer diamond, pink calcite, rhodonite, rose quartz.

About the plant Blue cypress is an evergreen tree with dark green leaves and cones, and reaches heights of up to 80 feet.

Chemical components Eudesmol, dihydrocolumellarin, guaiol, guaiazulene, chamazulene, columellarin, callitrin, cadalene, selinene, callitrisin, elemol.

Spiritual uses Blue cypress is an essential ingredient in synergetic blends used to facilitate shamanic journeys to the underworld. Heightening your consciousness and awareness, it is an excellent oil for lucid dreaming, journeywork, and vision seeking. Use this oil to improve your spiritual sight and clairvoyance. Cypress awakens in your consciousness a deeper understanding of your ancestors and improves your ability to commune with your loved ones on the Other Side.

Mental uses This oil grounds and calms the mind. The aroma of blue cypress activates and supports mental activity, stimulating creativity and the generation of new ideas.

Emotional uses In a synergistic blend with hyacinth essential oil, blue cypress nurtures and comforts during times of grief. It gives you the courage to turn to others for support while you allow your feelings of grief to take their normal course (which can be very rocky at times). It also supports and assists with the feelings, emotions, and self-acceptance associated with same-sex relationships. It aids in the transformational process of accepting yourself as you truly are and releasing potential judgments of others. This oil gives you strength as you experience an array of emotions—from guilt, anger, blame, shame, and confusion to relief, despair, betrayal, abandonment, and acceptance.

Physical uses Blue cypress relieves muscle and joint pain and relieves the symptoms of arthritis. Add it to a synergistic blend as a fixative to stabilize the scent of the volatile oils in a synergy. It is useful as an insect repellent. Some research indicates that it is helpful for the relief of allergies, insect bites, stings, and rashes. The antiviral properties assist in reducing the effects of pain and lessening the healing time of warts, cold sores, and shingles. Blue cypress is a good aromatherapy ally for artists, inventors, musicians, and writers.

Therapeutic properties Analgesic, antiarthritic, antibacterial, anti-inflammatory, antiviral, insecticidal, sedative.

Divine guidance Are you worried about how your loved ones who have passed away are doing on the Other Side? Are you concerned about people accepting you as you are? Be at peace and tell yourself, "My mind is calm and relaxed. I am sure my loved ones are safe and sound." Recognize that you have the ability to attract friends and associates who accept you exactly as you are. Tolerance and acceptance are part of your life—both in how you perceive others as well as how you are received.

For your safety Do not use if pregnant or nursing.

> **Interesting tidbits:**
> Cypress is a symbol of grief and mourning. It also has ties to the Underworld through the Greek legends of Kyparissos. Native Americans used cypress of Arizona for childbirth. Cypress is a perfumery note in Dior's *Poison*.

ELEMI
The Only Constant Is Change

BOTANICAL NAME	*Canarium luzonicum*
NOTE	top to middle
METHOD OF EXTRACTION	steam distillation
PARTS USED	gum or resin from bark
FRAGRANCE	citrusy, spicy
COLOR(S)	orange, yellow
CHAKRA(S)	navel, solar plexus, heart
ASTROLOGICAL SIGN(S)	Aquarius, Cancer
PLANET(S)	Moon, Uranus
NUMBER(S)	0, 5, 55
ANIMAL(S)	eagle, snake
ELEMENT(S)	air, water, fire

Affirmation I embrace change. I recognize that change can usher in improved life situations. I am grateful for the balanced movement of energy within me. I trust in the relaxed flow of the day. When I relax, great ideas jump into my consciousness.

Complementary flower essences Crab Apple to release toxins and habits. *Walnut* for dealing with change. *Wild Oat* to release perceived blocks.

Complementary stones Amber, ametrine, jet, lepidolite, orange calcite, smoky quartz.

About the plant Elemi is an evergreen tree that reaches heights of about 85 feet. It has fragrant yellow flowers that develop into plum-sized fruit containing the java almond.

Chemical components Limonene, elemol, phellandrene, elemicin, cymene, pinene, cineole, myrcene, sabinene, methyl eugenol.

Spiritual uses The calming effects of elemi make it a perfect aid for meditation. Inhale elemi to activate your intuition, along with a sense of assuredness. Elemi enhances psychic abilities. Use this oil with the intention of inviting sudden bursts of insight and "aha" moments for yourself and those around you during meditation or spiritual practice.

Mental uses Elemi improves your connection with the inner genius. Use this oil to incorporate good thoughts and positive thinking into your life. This essential oil encourages you to make the changes needed to restructure the thoughts that are constantly rotating through your consciousness. Let this oil be a reminder to observe the thoughts you have and to make sure those thoughts are what you want to broadcast to the universe! Whatever we think about becomes our reality.

Emotional uses Allow the vibration of elemi to assist you during times of change. Use it with the intention to allow the new to filter in as you release old emotions, fearful feelings, and belief systems that create perceived blocks. Elemi has the vibration for breaking free and change. Elemi helps you to detach from that which is no longer for your highest good, while maintaining a sense of calm and surrender during vulnerable times. Inhale this essential oil while you repeat the affirmations above. Elemi can help you get in touch with deep feelings and find healthy ways to communicate those feelings.

Physical uses Use elemi to encourage restful sleep. It is also helpful for reducing excessive perspiration, as well as for treating fungal infections and infected wounds. It reduces the production of mucus and is beneficial to deepening the breath, which is a good relaxation tool when releasing a smoking habit. It aids to calm the nerves during the process of becoming a nonsmoker. Deeply inhale fresh air with elemi diffused into the air as a replacement for inhaling cigarette smoke. Elemi can be used as a fixative for synergetic blends that include citrus oils. Elemi is a good aromatherapy ally for astrologers, clairvoyants, drug rehabilitation specialists, intuitive readers, meditation facilitators/practitioners, and neurologists.

Therapeutic properties Analgesic, antibacterial, antifungal, antiseptic, antitussive, antiviral, balsamic, cicatrizant, nervine, stimulative (immune system), stomachic, tonic, vulnerary.

Divine guidance Are you experiencing major changes in your life that are challenging your emotional state? Trust in the process of change and acknowledge and honor your feelings. Take the time to balance your physical, mental, emotional, and spiritual energy.

For your safety Do not use with young children. Do not use if pregnant or nursing.

> **Interesting tidbits:**
> Ancient Egyptians used elemi in the embalming process.

EUCALYPTUS
Breathe Deeply

BOTANICAL NAME	*Eucalyptus globulus* and *Eucalyptus radiata*
NOTE	top to middle
METHOD OF EXTRACTION	steam distillation
PARTS USED	leaves and twigs
FRAGRANCE	medicinal, penetrating, peppery, powerful, stimulating
COLOR(S)	blue, brown, green, gray
CHAKRA(S)	all
ASTROLOGICAL SIGN(S)	Aries, Gemini
PLANET(S)	Mars, Mercury
NUMBER(S)	5, 15, 55
ANIMAL(S)	koala, porcupine
ELEMENT(S)	air, earth

Affirmation I breathe deeply and oxygen replenishes my body. I feel protected. I am mindful of the energetic connections between others and myself. I automatically remove unhealthy cords of attachment that affect me mentally, emotionally, physically, and spiritually. Only goodness and love are allowed in my space. I am protected from negative influences.

Complementary flower essences Gentian to clear blocks and activate motivation. *Holly* to release anger and attract trustworthy people. *Walnut* to break unhealthy attachments and habits.

Complementary stones Black tourmaline, blue agate, blue chalcedony, chrysocolla, kambaba jasper, lapis lazuli, sodalite.

About the plant With aromatic green leaves and gray bark, *globulus* reaches a height of up to 480 feet, making it one of the world's tallest trees. With dark bark and narrow green aromatic leaves, *radiata* grows up to 170 feet tall.

Chemical components (*Globulus*) cineole, pinene, limonene, globulol, pinocarveol, cymene, aromadendrene, pinocarvone (*radiata*) cineole, terpineol piperitol, piperitone, geraniol, pinene, caryophyllene, terpinen, myrcene.

Spiritual uses Eucalyptus is a good essential oil to incorporate into your meditation or yoga practice since it helps you to be mindful of your breath and allows for clear respiratory passages as well as a clear mind. Eucalyptus is helpful for bringing forth the vibration of Archangel Michael and higher levels of protection. Eucalyptus clears negative psychic energy, so it's a good oil to add to a synergistic blend to clear the energetic space.

Mental uses Eucalyptus increases cerebral blood flow, which is why it increases alertness. It is beneficial when you are setting the intention to release negative or toxic thoughts. The refreshing scent activates a cleansing of the mental processes that are creating perceived blocks.

Emotional uses Eucalyptus has a cooling quality if you are feeling hotheaded and angry. Inhale eucalyptus deeply to release feelings of agitation and frustration. Use it in an aromatic-energetic mist to shift the energy of a room and cleanse it of intense emotions.

Physical uses Use eucalyptus at the first sign of a cold or respiratory challenge to reduce or release the symptoms of cold, flu, and allergies. It opens up all breathing passages to relieve congestion of nose, sinus, and bronchial airways. Eucalyptus is helpful for relieving painful, aching muscles.

Eucalyptus radiata helps relieve the pain and symptoms of shingles (herpes zoster). It is an excellent deodorizer for your body as well as for the air. It is also a very good disinfectant. Eucalyptus radiata is one of the best natural insect repellents, said to work for up to 90 minutes. Eucalyptus, both radiata and globulus, is a good aromatherapy ally for athletes, environmentalists, housekeepers, infectious disease specialists, law enforcement professionals, marathon participants, pest control professionals, and pulmonary specialists.

Therapeutic properties Analgesic, antibacterial, antibiotic, antidiabetic, antidote, antifungal, anti-inflammatory, antineuralgic, antiparasitic, antipruritic, antiputrid, antirheumatic, antiseptic (strong), antispasmodic, antitussive, antivenomous, antiviral (respiratory tract), astringent, cephalic, cicatrizant, cooling, decongestant, deodorizer, depurative, diaphoretic, diuretic, febrifugal, germicide, hemostatic, insecticidal, invigorating, purifying, regenerative (skin tissue), rubefacient, stimulative (circulatory system), tonic, uplifting, vulnerary.

Divine guidance Have you been experiencing too much negative energy from others as well as yourself? Do you get frequent headaches or sinus conditions? Steps to restore emotional, physical, and mental balance are in order. Try visualization, meditation, and/or aromatherapy to bring a new calmness to every aspect of your life and body. Peace and tranquility are always available to you.

For your safety Avoid (or use small amounts) if epileptic or in cases of high blood pressure. May interfere with efficacy of homeopathic remedies. Do not use if pregnant or nursing. Avoid use on children.

Interesting tidbits:

Eucalyptus essential oil is commonly used in saunas and spas. The leaves of the eucalyptus tree are the koala's only food. Use to eliminate dust mites on beds and fabrics. Eucalyptus radiata is one of the ingredients in my Auntie M's blends.

FENNEL
Smooth Transitions

Botanical name	*Foeniculum vulgare*
Note	middle to top
Method of extraction	steam distillation
Parts used	seeds
Fragrance	herbaceous, licorice-like, powdery, sweet
Color(s)	green, olive green, chartreuse green, yellow
Chakra(s)	solar plexus
Astrological sign(s)	Cancer, Gemini, Virgo
Planet(s)	Earth, Mercury, Moon
Number(s)	40/4
Animal(s)	porcupine, sloth, spider
Element(s)	air, water

Affirmation I am interested in the world around me. I enjoy life and my strong sense of purpose. Even when the world around me is constantly changing, I remain grounded and focused. I tap into the innate healing abilities to realign my emotional, spiritual, and physical bodies.

Complementary flower essences Agrimony to release mental torment and find genuine happiness. *Clematis* to help you stay present and to fulfill your creative potential. *Walnut* to deal with natural changes and cycles of life. *White Chestnut* to release unwanted thoughts and memories.

Complementary stones Apatite, citrine, citron chrysoprase, chrysoprase, golden calcite, green calcite, peridot, prehnite.

About the plant Native to Asia and Europe, fennel grows in stalks about 3–7 feet high and is similar in appearance to celery. It has green hairlike leaves and yellow flowers that turn to seed.

Chemical components Anethole, limonene, fenchone, estragole, pinene, phellandrene.

Spiritual uses Fennel encourages tolerance, compassion, and understanding. Use this oil to raise your awareness with the intention of observing yourself or a situation from a higher perspective. Fennel helps keep a clean filter for channeling and accessing the Akashic Records (information and records of all that has ever been, all that will ever be, and the unlimited potential realities stored in nonphysical space available to everyone).

Mental uses Fennel helps increase your courage and allows you to foresee the results of your actions in your mind's eye. Fennel aids in increasing mental strength to deal with repetitive or unwanted thoughtforms and helps let go of worries and unhappy memories. Use fennel with the intention to stop mentally reliving arguments or agitating scenarios. With its stress-reducing properties, it also helps you to realize what you can do to absorb and process life with more ease.

Emotional uses Fennel helps you process emotional aggravation that manifests as indigestion, heartburn, or an upset stomach, helping you to look more objectively at what feelings, people, places, and situations are causing you agitation. On an emotional level, it helps process or deal with the source of the aggravation. Inhale the sweet scent of fennel to help garner the courage to clear away blocks and to fulfill your life agreements.

Physical uses Fennel helps relieve water retention and inflammation. Use it to aid your body in the release of excess fat as well. Fennel relieves flatulence and aids with digestion, specifically with the proper functioning of the gallbladder, liver, pancreas, spleen, and kidneys—and the proper production of digestive enzymes. Fennel is helpful for relieving menstrual pain and tension. Due to the estragole chemical constituent, it may affect hormones by having an estrogen-like effect. It is known to improve lactation in nursing mothers when used in moderation. Fennel is a good aromatherapy ally for dieticians, doulas, gastroenterologists, and gynecologists.

Therapeutic properties Antibacterial, antidotal, antiemetic, antifungal, antiparasitic, antiphlogistic, antiseptic, antispasmodic, antitoxic, antitussive, aperitive, astringent, calmative, carminative, decongestant, depurative, detoxifier, diaphoretic, digestive, diuretic, emmenagogic, estrogenic, galactagogic, hepatic, insecticidal, laxative, regulator (female reproductive system), resolvent, revitalizing, stimulative (uterine contractions, estrogen levels), stomachic, tonic.

Divine guidance What is it about life that you just can't swallow? Are you challenged by people or situations that agitate you? Are you having a hard time sorting out all the details of what's going on around you and within you? Do you need to gain some understanding to get clear on what direction you want to head? It is time to take a grounded approach and gather realistic solutions by taking the necessary time to examine yourself and the situation through quiet contemplation.

For your safety May inhibit blood clotting, so avoid if on anticoagulants. Avoid if prone to epileptic seizures. Avoid use if pregnant or nursing. If used for lactation, use in moderation.

> **Interesting tidbits:**
> Fennel seeds are often used in traditional Italian tomato sauce recipes. Historically, fennel is believed to avert the evil eye.

FRANKINCENSE
The Wise Ones

BOTANICAL NAME	*Boswellia carteri*
NOTE	base to middle
METHOD OF EXTRACTION	steam distillation
PARTS USED	resin of tree
FRAGRANCE	balsamic, dry, resinous, rich, sweet, woody; reminiscent of a museum of fine art or a church
COLOR(S)	magenta, purple, white
CHAKRA(S)	crown, third eye, heart
ASTROLOGICAL SIGN(S)	Aquarius, Pisces
PLANET(S)	Uranus, Venus
NUMBER(S)	11, 22, 33, 44
ANIMAL(S)	all animals, but especially elephants
ELEMENT(S)	air, fire

Affirmation I focus on empathy and kindness. Each day, my intention is to live, love, and act with compassion and tolerance toward every person I encounter. I am aligned with the healing powers of inner peace and kindness. I am able to help others by vibrating love through my presence, words, and actions.

Complementary flower essences Elm for feelings of depression and to increase confidence and focus. *White Chestnut* to release the incessant chatter in your mind. *Wild Oat* to realize your life purpose.

Complementary stones Amethyst, green apophyllite, magenta-dyed agate, purple-dyed agate, kyanite.

About the plant Native to the hot, dry climate of the Mediterranean, frankincense is a small tree that reaches a height of about 20 feet.

Chemical components Alpha-pinene, limonene, sabinene, myrcene, beta-caryophyllene, alpha-thujene, para-cymene.

Spiritual uses Frankincense is the ultimate oil for meditation practice. It helps you to align yourself with compassion, inner peace, tolerance, and love. Frankincense aligns you with higher consciousness. It increases your awareness of the spiritual and mystical experience of the unity of the universe. The unity of this higher consciousness is also called superconsciousness (Yoga), objective consciousness (Gurdjieff), Buddhic consciousness (Theosophy), cosmic consciousness, God-consciousness (Sufism and Hinduism), and Christ Consciousness (New Thought). This is a perfect oil for spiritual counselors, intuitive readers, keynote speakers, Reiki practitioners, and meditation facilitators. Use it to align with Archangel Zaphkiel (Tzaphkiel) for understanding and mindfulness and with Archangel Uriel for illumination and peace.

Mental uses Use frankincense to clear your mind of incessant chatter. The result is clarity of consciousness. Allow the scent of frankincense to automatically translate thoughts and feelings to a deeper understanding of yourself. Frankincense brings higher levels of clarity to life's experiences and can help you to quickly center yourself and quiet your thoughts. Use it for focus and grounding.

Emotional uses Frankincense brings a sense of calm and inner peace, thereby quieting ruffled emotions and out-of-balance feelings. As frankincense facilitates deep breathing, it also aids in calming hysteria. Inhale frankincense in a synergistic blend with bergamot, lemon, sweet marjoram, and other oils to ease feelings of anxiousness and the symptoms of depression. In *The Fragrant*

Mind, Worwood states that frankincense aids to heal addiction, aggression, fear of change, facing death, letting go, forgiveness, grief, and panic attacks.

Physical uses Use frankincense for all respiratory concerns. It is beneficial for opening breathing passages. It's perfect for the healing process during recovery of pneumonia, pleurisy, bronchitis, sinus congestion, and similar ailments. Frankincense fortifies the immune system, and it has been found to be beneficial for relief from arthritis. Frankincense is a good aromatherapy ally for acupuncturists, healthcare practitioners, life coaches, mystics, pulmonary specialists, spiritual counselors, intuitive readers, keynote speakers, Reiki practitioners, and meditation facilitators/practitioners.

Therapeutic properties Abortifacient, analgesic, antibacterial, antibiotic, antidepressant, anti-inflammatory, antioxidant, antiseptic, antispasmodic, antitussive, astringent, carminative, cephalic, cicatrizant, cytophylactic, digestive, diuretic, emmenagogic, emollient, fixative, nervine, purgative, rejuvenator (skin), revitalizing, sedative, stimulative (cells, immune system), tonic, tonifying (skin), uplifting, vulnerary, warming.

Divine guidance Do you wish to gain clearer insight or a better understanding of a situation? Make an appointment with yourself to meditate or sit in silence. Do this often. Open your consciousness and listen for your soul's truth and embrace it without judgment. Mental clarity and self-acceptance are the gifts of a regular meditation practice.

For your safety No known contraindications.

> **Interesting tidbits:**
> Frankincense has been a valued resin for over 5,000 years. Ancient Egyptians used the crushed, charred remains of burned frankincense, called *kohl,* as eyeliner. This resin is traditionally associated with the Three Wise Men, who are believed by some historians to have been Zoroastrian astrologer-priests from Babylon. One of their gifts to the infant Jesus the Christ was frankincense.

GERANIUM
Restorative Balance

BOTANICAL NAME	*Pelargonium graveolens*
NOTE	middle
METHOD OF EXTRACTION	steam distillation
PARTS USED	leaves
FRAGRANCE	floral, fresh, sweet, fruity, strong
COLOR(S)	blue, orange, turquoise
CHAKRA(S)	navel
ASTROLOGICAL SIGN(S)	Cancer, Scorpio
PLANET(S)	Jupiter, Moon, Venus
NUMBER(S)	8
ANIMAL(S)	snake
ELEMENT(S)	water, earth

Affirmation My body is in a constant state of restoration and healing. I find balance in my life through play, work, rest, exercise, and laughter. I easily nurture myself. I have constant protection surrounding me, which deflects anything that is not for my highest good.

Complementary flower essences Cherry Plum to maintain control and composure. *Holly* to calm anger and aggression. *Impatiens* for patience with yourself and others.

Complementary stones Azurite-malachite, bloodstone, carnelian, chrysocolla, lapis lazuli, rhodonite, sodalite.

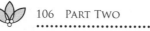

About the plant Geranium is a small, fragrant plant with brilliantly colored flowers and grows to a height of about 3 feet. It is a genus of 422 species.

Chemical components Citronellol, geraniol, linalool, citronellyl formate, isomenthone, eudesmol, geranyl formate, geranyl butyrate, geranyl tiglate, caryophyllene, guaia, germacrene D, geranyl propionate, rose oxide, phenylethyl butyrate.

Spiritual uses Geranium is beneficial for personal transformation. Geranium invokes guardians of protection, keeping away negative energy. Use geranium oil to connect with the spiritual power of the sun as a source of nourishment for your soul and the moon for understanding life cycles. This oil is ideal for connecting with Archangel Raphael to restore and rejuvenate on all levels and Archangel Sabrael to deter jealousy and negative forces.

Mental uses Geranium helps maintain focus on something important when your thoughts are scattered. Its calming effect helps you sort out thoughts. By making it your intention to change your mind, geranium helps cancel out angry, vindictive, or negative thoughts. It is helpful to inhale this essential oil while you repeat the affirmations above.

Emotional uses Use geranium to rebalance yourself while you are experiencing hormonal havoc. Allow yourself to remember your realizations, feelings, and the subject of righteous indignation during this period and let the geranium assist in gently sorting out these profound emotions. Geranium is helpful for relieving the symptoms of postpartum depression. Geranium is helpful when you are going through times of higher-than-normal irritability and crying episodes.

Physical uses Geranium is beneficial in the treatment of mouth ulcers and reduces inflammation of the mucous membranes of the mouth. It also relieves itching and swelling of hemorrhoids. Geranium is effective to aid in hormonal balance. Use this oil in a synergistic blend with clary sage and lavender to create stability in menstrual cycles, to assist in fertility, and for relief of

PMS symptoms and hot flashes. Geranium has been known to aid in clearing endometriosis. Massage geranium in combination with lavender, bergamot, and chamomile in a carrier oil to reduce cellulite and increase circulation. Add geranium to a natural insect repellent blend along with eucalyptus and lavender. It is effective for the treatment of insect bites, spider bites, and wasp stings. Geranium is an aromatherapy ally for dental professionals, doulas, gynecologists, law enforcement professionals, marriage counselors, massage therapists, mothers, and phlebotomists.

Therapeutic properties Analgesic, antibacterial, antibiotic, anticoagulative, antidepressant, antidiabetic, antifungal, anti-inflammatory, antineuralgic, antiseptic, antispasmodic, antistress, astringent, antiparasitic, cicatrizant, cytophylactic, deodorizer, depurative, diuretic, healing, hemostatic, insecticidal, regulator (glandular functions and hormones), rejuvenator (skin tissue), sedative (mild) (anxiety), stimulative (adrenal glands; circulatory and lymphatic systems), tonic, tonifying (skin), uplifting (menopause and premenstrual tension), vasoconstrictor, vulnerary.

Divine guidance Are you dealing with an inflamed or unbalanced situation—physically, mentally, spiritually, or emotionally? Have you been challenged by imbalances in your body? Take steps to balance your emotions through journaling, exercise, and healthy communication. It is important to reestablish your equilibrium—physically, mentally, and emotionally—after periods of intensity.

For your safety Do not use if pregnant, although it can be helpful during labor and delivery if prescribed by a reputable healthcare practitioner.

Interesting tidbits:

Geranium is said to bring blessings of friendship and good relationships. Offering a variety of colors, scents, and leaf patterns, geraniums have been a favorite in American gardens for more than 200 years. Place potted geraniums outside the front door of your home to welcome in good energy and detract negativity.

GINGER
Vim and Vigor

BOTANICAL NAME	*Zingiber officinale*
NOTE	middle to base
METHOD OF EXTRACTION	steam distillation
PARTS USED	rhizome and roots
FRAGRANCE	lemony, spicy, pungent, warm, woody subsidiary notes
COLOR(S)	orange, yellow, red
CHAKRA(S)	root, navel, solar plexus, heart
ASTROLOGICAL SIGN(S)	Cancer, Virgo
PLANET(S)	Juno, Pallas Athena, Mercury, Moon
NUMBER(S)	10
ANIMAL(S)	hummingbird
ELEMENT(S)	fire

Affirmation I have the strength to do anything I set out to do with loving intention. Vital life force flows vibrantly through me. My energy abounds. I'm self-motivated to be productive. My tasks and creative projects are completed with ease. I am grateful for my energetic passion for life!

Complementary flower essences Oak to help you allow time to renew and rejuvenate. *Gentian* to restore confidence and motivation. *Hornbeam* to activate energy and enthusiasm.

Complementary stones Ruby, rhodochrosite, rhodonite, garnet, carnelian, honey calcite, orange calcite, golden calcite.

About the plant Found in tropical and subtropical climates, ginger has lance-like leaves and typically reaches heights of up to 4 feet. It has white, yellow, pink, or red flowers and thick rhizomes.

Chemical components Zingiberene, alpha-selinene, beta-sesquiphellandrene, delta-cadinene, beta-phellandrene, cineol, limonene, curcumene.

Spiritual uses Ginger's spicy aroma is a stimulant for awakening consciousness. It clears away the energetic cobwebs, opening portals of awareness to receive insights and information. Ginger has the energetics to strengthen your energy field on many levels. Add ginger to a synergistic blend with the intention of activating your intuitive skills. Use ginger in synergetic blends with other oils like frankincense, grapefruit, and vetiver for channeling and meditation to align with Maha Chohan (an Ascended Master director with the strength and dedication to hold the vision and intention to activate the Divine Spark in humankind) as well as with memories of the pure teachings of Atlantis.

Mental uses Ginger is helpful for increasing motivation, relieving apathy, and aiding in the decision-making process. Ginger helps you remember that you have the power to create and transform your reality with your mind. It improves willpower and clarity. It can invigorate your mind and improve your memory.

Emotional uses Ginger helps to defrost frozen emotions and feelings of coldness toward others. It helps open your emotional field to accept connection with other people as well as a romantic relationship. In some cultures, ginger has been used as an aphrodisiac. It promotes courage and confidence and is an excellent aid for balancing the solar plexus chakra.

Physical uses Ginger is especially good for relieving nausea and is helpful for digestion. Use ginger in a synergistic blend to relieve congestion, coughs, colds, and flu. This root has been used as an antidote to poison. It is an overall stimulant and catalytic, which maximizes the effectiveness of a remedy or blend. Ginger is helpful for relieving inflammation and pain. Use it in synergistic blends for uncomfortable menstrual symptoms, stomach discomfort, headaches, or just as an overall tonic to rejuvenate your body. Ginger is a good aromatherapy ally for actors, fertility specialists, herbalists, leaders, marriage counselors, mystics, sex therapists, and travel professionals.

Therapeutic properties Analgesic, antiparasitic, antibacterial, anticoagulant, antiemetic, anti-inflammatory, antioxidant, antiscorbutic, antiseptic, antispasmodic, antitoxic, antitussive, aperitive, aphrodisiac, astringent (stops bleeding), carminative, cephalic, diaphoretic, digestive (nausea), diuretic, emmenagogic, febrifugal, laxative, rubefacient, stimulative (circulatory and nervous systems), stomachic, tonic, tonifying (digestive system).

Divine guidance Do you need more vitality, endurance, and pizazz? Are you experiencing overall congestion in your physical body—either on a respiratory or on a digestive level? Is your mind a bit foggy? It's time to clear your energy on all levels and get your vim and vigor recharged. Allow the old to be released and let the new in. It is time to take steps to improve your endurance and overall health. Get your energy centers recharged and renew your passion for living a vibrant life!

For your safety Possible skin irritant. Do not use if pregnant or nursing.

> **Interesting tidbits:**
> Ginger has been used for thousands of years. Hippocrates used it medicinally, Romans cooked with it, and the Chinese used it to make tea. In perfumery, ginger offers an Oriental flair. Its scent is predominant in Gucci's *Envy for Men*.

GRAPEFRUIT
Can You Hear the Angels Sing?

BOTANICAL NAME	*Citrus paradisi*
NOTE	top
METHOD OF EXTRACTION	cold-press
PARTS USED	fruit peel
FRAGRANCE	citrusy, floral, fresh, green, sweet
COLOR(S)	white, cobalt blue, pink, purple, yellow
CHAKRA(S)	crown, heart, solar plexus
ASTROLOGICAL SIGN(S)	Gemini, Leo, Virgo
PLANET(S)	Mercury, Sun
NUMBER(S)	33, 44, 444
ANIMAL(S)	dragonfly, fox, sloth
ELEMENT(S)	air, fire

Affirmation It is safe for me to shine my light brightly. I am self-confident and poised. I recognize my self-worth and step into my personal power with grace and ease. My internal brilliance shines through as I step forward into my life with the courage to be all that I can be! I am grateful for the guidance I receive from the angels who help orchestrate my life.

Complementary flower essences Cerato for guidance and self-confidence. *Gentian* to feel encouraged. *Larch* for confidence. *Mimulus* for courage. *Wild Oat* for direction and inner knowing. *Willow* to think positively.

Complementary stones Apache tears, apophyllite, clear quartz, citrine, danburite, golden calcite, golden topaz, kyanite, kunzite, rhodochrosite, rhodonite, rose quartz, unakite.

About the plant Grapefruit is a fruit-bearing evergreen tree that reaches a height of about 15 to 25 feet.

Chemical components Limonene, myrcene, pinene, sabinene, nootkatone.

Spiritual uses Grapefruit has a high vibration that helps you raise your consciousness and awareness to receive messages from angels, archangels, and master guides. Use this oil to connect with Saint Germain and the Archangels Camael, Jophiel, Metatron, and Michael. This essential oil assists in bringing back good memories and the pure teachings of Atlantis.

Mental uses Grapefruit oil sharpens memory and mental clarity. With its mind-clearing properties, this oil is beneficial when writing or working on detailed tasks that require focus, all the while bringing more joy to the project. Inhale this essential oil while you repeat the affirmations above.

Emotional uses Grapefruit essential oil, especially the pink variety, helps to open your heart to receive blessings, joy, and happiness. It evokes feelings of bliss and comfort, as if supportive, kindred spirits surround you. Use this oil to help develop a stronger sense of self and to rid your emotional body of doubt and fear. Trust that you can develop loving relationships with this oil in your energy field. Use grapefruit to return to joy after periods of grief.

Physical uses Due to its purifying nature, grapefruit balances body fluids and stimulates the lymphatic system. Grapefruit has a cleansing effect on the kidneys and is a diuretic. It is helpful as a weight-loss aid for digestion of fats. Grapefruit essential oil is a good addition to a blend for the intention of reducing cellulite. Add to a synergistic blend to improve physical strength and vitality. Grapefruit is a good aromatherapy ally for accountants, angel communicators, aromatherapists, authors, dieticians, editors, hospice care-givers, intuitive readers, leaders, massage therapists, neurologists, nutrition-ists, and weight-loss/weight-gain counselors.

Therapeutic properties Antibacterial, antidepressant, antiseptic, an-tistress, antitoxic, antiviral, aperitive, astringent, balancing (central nervous system), cephalic, cholagogic, depurative, detoxifier, digestive, diuretic, hemostatic, resolvent, restorative, reviving, stimulative (digestive and lym-phatic systems, and neurotransmitters), tonic (liver), tonifying (skin).

Divine guidance Have you noticed that you are very intuitive lately? Are you listening to your inner guidance? Listen to that still, small voice within to find the answers you seek. It is time to gain clarity and have a clearer picture of what is truly going on within you and around you. Can you see the bigger picture? Get focused and stay focused! Take the time to meditate and try to see the greater perspective from varying points of view.

For your safety This oil is phototoxic; therefore, avoid exposure to direct sunlight when using topically.

> ### Interesting tidbits:
> Grapefruit essential oil is derived from either white or pink grapefruit varieties. The oil from pink grapefruit has a slightly sweeter fragrance, which creates a higher top note. The majority of the synergistic blends I create for higher spiritual alignment "want" grapefruit as part of the formula to raise the vibration.

HELICHRYSUM
Blessings from Heaven and Earth

BOTANICAL NAME	*Helichrysum angustifolium*
NOTE	base
METHOD OF EXTRACTION	steam distillation
PARTS USED	flowers
FRAGRANCE	earthy, floral, green, sweet
COLOR(S)	green, white, yellow
CHAKRA(S)	crown, heart, solar plexus
ASTROLOGICAL SIGN(S)	Libra, Scorpio
PLANET(S)	Pluto, Venus
NUMBER(S)	22, 33, 44
ANIMAL(S)	eagle, hawk, owl, unicorn
ELEMENT(S)	air, water

Affirmation All that I need is always within my reach. I am grateful for all that I have. I accept the impermanent nature of life. I easily adapt to my changing environment. Change is good. I embrace transitions as they exist within life. I give love to others and readily accept theirs in return. I relax in nature to regenerate and rejuvenate.

Complementary flower essences Red Chestnut to relieve stress and worry about the welfare of others. *Sweet Chestnut* for inner strength. *Walnut* to aid during times of change.

Complementary stones Honey calcite, Isis quartz point, jet, lapis lazuli, morganite, peridot, rhodochrosite, rhodonite, rose quartz.

About the plant Helichrysum is a flower plant of the daisy family that grows to a height of approximately 2 feet with yellow flowers. There are about 500 species of helichrysum.

Chemical components Pinene, curcumene, neryl acetate, selinene, italidione I, caryophyllene, curcumene, italicene, selinene, caryophyllene oxide, limonene, selina, italidone III, capaene, isoitalicene, bergamotene.

Spiritual uses Helichrysum is an oil used for anointing during ceremonies focused on entering and exiting this planet. Use it for baby blessings and for those who are transitioning from this earthly existence. Because of its relaxing properties it is beneficial for meditation and almost any type of spiritual ceremony. Helichrysum helps improve your spiritual sight and knowing (clairvoyance and claircognizance). Use it to help spirits and disincarnate entities find their way to the Light or the Other Side.

Mental uses Helichrysum is a stress reliever. Use this to improve overall outlook on life and positive perspective. Helichrysum is beneficial when you are going through a rite of passage or ritual. This oil helps you transcend any challenge presented through inner strength, connection to higher realms of consciousness, and Divine will. It also assists you in thinking outside the box by opening your mind to unlimited possibilities.

Emotional uses Helichrysum supports you through any kind of transition. It is especially helpful for hospice caregivers and the loved ones of a family member as they transition to the Other Side. Use this essential oil when there is a conflict between your emotions and your common sense. It helps you accept when old friends depart your life and new alliances and networks form.

Physical uses Helichrysum promotes cell regeneration and rejuvenation and aids in the healing of scars and wounds. Use helichrysum for aches and pains, including the discomforts associated with PMS and menopause. Helichrysum has been used for asthma, bronchitis, and whooping cough as well as migraine, headaches, and skin problems, according to Julia Lawless in *The Encyclopedia of Essential Oils*. Due to its strong purification properities, use helichrysum for detoxification from drugs, alcohol, or nicotine. It is an aromatherapy ally for doulas, drug counselors, estheticians, hospice workers, ministers, and spiritual counselors.

Therapeutic properties Analgesic, antibacterial, anticoagulant, antidepressant, antifungal, anti-inflammatory, antiseptic, antispasmodic, antitussive, antiviral, astringent, cephalic, cholagogic, cicatrizant, cytophylactic, detoxifier, diuretic, hepatic, nervine, sedative, tonic.

Divine guidance Do you treat yourself well? What kind of self-talk is going on in your mind? Are you trying to change your life? Start by changing the way you look at things. Open your mind to the unlimited possibilities of the seen and the unseen. You are a visionary. Use your intuitive skills to open up your potential realities. This is a time to pay attention to how well you treat yourself and to be aware of your inner chatter so that you can make necessary changes. It is time to awaken your consciousness fully and to focus on love for yourself and all beings.

For your safety No known contraindications.

> **Interesting tidbits:**
> Helichrysum is also known as immortelle. *Immortelle* means "everlasting" in French. It is used in beauty creams for wrinkle reduction, including L'Occitane's Immortelle Precious Cream.

HYACINTH
Comfort: This Too Shall Pass

BOTANICAL NAME	*Hyacinthus orientalis*
NOTE	top
METHOD OF EXTRACTION	solvent extraction
PARTS USED	flowers
FRAGRANCE	deep, exotic, floral, green, heady, sweet, soft
COLOR(s)	white, pink, purple
CHAKRA(s)	crown, heart, third eye
ASTROLOGICAL SIGN(s)	Aquarius, Pisces, Libra
PLANET(s)	Neptune, Pluto, Venus
NUMBER(s)	11, 22
ANIMAL(s)	bear, raven
ELEMENT(s)	air, water

Affirmation I know that intense feelings of anger, sorrow, and grief will pass. I release resentment and rage from my body, mind, and spirit. I open myself up to the healing energy of the love and prayers being sent my way.

Complementary flower essences Cherry Plum to help maintain composure. *Mimulus* for courage. *Star of Bethlehem* for comfort and relief from feelings of trauma. *Walnut* to deal with the changes and cycles of life. *White Chestnut* to help you switch off repetitive thoughts.

Complementary stones Amethyst druzy (spirit quartz), Apache tears, apophyllite, citrine, danburite, kunzite, rhodochrosite, rhodonite, rose quartz, unakite.

About the plant Hyacinth is a small plant that grows to a height of 6–8 inches tall, with slender green leaves and fragrant pink, purple, or white bell-shaped flowers that, when open fully, look like starfish.

Chemical components Benzyl alcohol, cinnamyl alcohol, benzyl acetate, benzyl benzoate, phenylethanol, trimethoxybenzene, methyleugenol, phenylethyl benzoate, methoxyphenylethanol.

Spiritual uses Hyacinth is ideal for activating the energy field that connects you to the spirit realm, facilitating your connection with loved ones on the Other Side who can act as spirit guides. Use the oil to tune in to the cosmic forces of the Universe, providing you with a direct link to wisdom and knowledge. Draw on the energy of hyacinth in meditation practice and use it with the intention to communicate with Ascended Masters like Saint Germain and other teachers of the higher realm.

Mental uses Hyacinth relieves stress and tension. Its sweet scent helps transform negative thought patterns to positive thoughtforms. It's especially beneficial during the grieving process to shift sad thoughts to happy, nostalgic memories. Hyacinth helps improve self-esteem through positive self-talk and awakening of the realization of your personal magnificence.

Emotional uses Using hyacinth for comfort during the grieving process goes back as far as ancient Egypt. This essential oil is helpful during all phases and types of grief, whether it is the loss of a loved one, friendship or relationship, career, or any loss-related emotional challenge. This essential oil helps to relieve raw feelings of heartache. Inhale this essential oil while you repeat the affirmations above to release resentment and allow for forgiveness. It opens your heart to understanding how to truly release past challenges.

Physical uses Hyacinth is primarily used in perfumery. Its health benefits are derived from the emotional release of potentially poisonous feelings such as resentment, anger, grief, and extreme sadness, thereby promoting over-all well-being. Hyacinth is a good aromatherapy ally for clairvoyants, spiritual counselors, grief counselors, hospice caregivers, mystics, and sex therapists.

Therapeutic properties Antidepressant, antiseptic, aphrodisiac, hypnotic, sedative.

Divine guidance Are you in the process of healing after the loss of a job, relationship, pet, or loved one? It is important to reestablish your equilibrium—physically, mentally, and emotionally—after periods of intensity. Try this: Look in the mirror, smile, and say, "I love you!" It's time to cultivate a deeper relationship with yourself. Uncover what you can do for yourself to increase your happiness.

For your safety No known contraindications.

> **Interesting tidbits:**
> In ancient Egypt, hyacinth was used to aid with the grieving process. Pure hyacinth essential oil as a single note is rare. This is a good alternative to synthetically fragranced oil, as it has a beautiful, sweet, floral, green, and honey-like aroma.

HYSSOP
Breathe Deeply

BOTANICAL NAME	*Hyssopus officinalis*
NOTE	middle
METHOD OF EXTRACTION	steam distillation
PARTS USED	leaves and flowers
FRAGRANCE	warm, sweet
COLOR(S)	black, brown, gray, orange
CHAKRA(S)	crown, root
ASTROLOGICAL SIGN(S)	Scorpio
PLANET(S)	Chiron, Mars, Pluto
NUMBER(S)	8
ANIMAL(S)	dog, dragon, spider
ELEMENT(S)	fire, water

Affirmation It is easy for me to rise above challenging situations. I am grateful for life experiences to help me grow and evolve. I am safe and sound. As I breathe deeply and fully, I know all is well. I am divinely protected.

Complementary flower essences Rock Rose to feel safe and protected. *Star of Bethlehem* to rebalance after shock. *Willow* for forgiveness.

Complementary stones Amethyst, black tourmaline, gold tiger's eye, red tiger's eye, rhodonite, tiger iron.

About the plant Hyssop is a bushy plant that grows to 1–2 feet tall with narrow aromatic leaves and blue, dark purple, pink, or white flowers.

Chemical components Linalool, cineole, limonene, pinene, caryo-phyllene oxide, camphene, myrcene, isopinocamphone, bourbonene, sabinene, pinocamphone.

Spiritual uses Hyssop oil is useful in a synergistic blend for cleansing and purification rituals. Hyssop helps when you need to rise above challenging situations to grasp the higher purpose of life experiences. Hyssop has been used in formulas for psychic self-defense and can be used to clear your home of negative vibrations. It adds a layer of protection when spread around the perimeter of a home or at the entry points of a building. Hyssop assists in the grieving process, specifically in helping you release that which no longer serves your highest good.

Mental uses In very small quantities, hyssop amplifies a synergistic blend to help you release your own negative thinking. Use this oil for contemplation to examine your own thoughts and beliefs in order to release those that no longer serve you. Use this oil to help purify your thoughts and, therefore, your life. Hyssop also stimulates creativity.

Emotional uses Hyssop brings in a sense of calm and relieves anxiety. It helps you release resentment in situations in which forgiveness is needed by helping you to maintain a sense of gratitude for the experience's role in your personal development. Hyssop heightens the awareness that your own thinking is what has the power to create the most challenging life circumstances; through self-acceptance and the release of sorrow over the situation, the emotional body can be brought back into balance.

Physical uses Hyssop helps improve breathing by opening the sinuses and alleviating the symptoms of asthma, bronchitis, coughs, and colds. It also helps relieve digestion and gas. Hyssop oil can regulate the menstrual cycle. Its diuretic properties help reduce water retention, but be aware as it also raises blood pressure. Hyssop is a good aromatherapy ally for artists, judges, law enforcement professionals, and pulmonary specialists.

Therapeutic properties Antibacterial, anti-inflammatory, antirheumatic, antiseptic, antispasmodic, antitussive, antiparasitic, antiviral, astringent, balsamic, cardiac, carminative, cephalic, cicatrizant, depurative, diaphoretic, digestive, diuretic, emmenagogic, emollient, febrifugal, hypertensor, laxative (mild), nervine, regulatory (blood pressure), resolvent, stimulative (adrenal glands), stomachic, sudorific, tonic, vulnerary.

Divine guidance Are you ready to slay the inner dragon and align with joy, health, and prosperity? Who do you need to forgive? It's time to release the congestion of your body and your mind, and open to breathe in life fully and completely. Aspire to reach the highest potential and use your inner strength to overcome obstacles appearing to be created by others. Go within and know the truth.

For your safety Use in small amounts and only if prescribed by a reputable healthcare practitioner or aromatherapist. Avoid in cases of high blood pressure. Do not use if pregnant or nursing.

> **Interesting tidbits:**
> Hyssop has been used for centuries in protection spells as well as in purification baths to overcome a bad habit or to counteract a jinx. Psalm 51:7 reads: "Purify me with hyssop, and I will be clean. Wash me, and I will be whiter than snow."

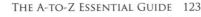

JASMINE
Blessings and Love

BOTANICAL NAME	*Jasminum grandiflorum*
NOTE	middle to base
METHOD OF EXTRACTION	solvent extraction
PARTS USED	flower petals
FRAGRANCE	green, floral, sweet
COLOR(S)	coral, pink, peach, white, yellow
CHAKRA(S)	crown, heart
ASTROLOGICAL SIGN(S)	Libra, Scorpio
PLANET(S)	Juno, Moon, Pluto, Venus
NUMBER(S)	7, 11
ANIMAL(S)	dove, rabbit
ELEMENT(S)	air

Affirmation I am blessed with nurturing vibrations wherever I go. I am gentle with myself. I enjoy loving relationships. I focus on all my good attributes and amplify them. I have the courage to step forward with joy and enthusiasm. I allow love into my life.

Complementary flower essences *Clematis* to be truly present with family and friends. *Honeysuckle* to feel grateful for this moment and a happy future. *Water Violet* to maintain a stronger connection with others. *Willow* to attract positive people into your life.

Complementary stones Apophyllite, carnelian, clear quartz, danburite, golden topaz, kunzite, moonstone, pink calcite, rhodochrosite, rose quartz, selenite.

About the plant Jasmine is a shrub native to Asia that reaches heights of up to 40 feet. It has aromatic white flowers.

Chemical components Benzyl acetate, benzyl benzoate, phytol, squalene, isophytol, phytyl acetate, linalool, geranyl linalool, indole, jasmine, eugenol, methyl jasmonate, jasmolactone, methyl benzoate.

Spiritual uses Use jasmine oil to call upon Archangel Auriel to assist in the realignment of the Divine Feminine and alleviate subconscious fears. You can also use this oil to call upon Saint Therese of Lisieux to help manifest miracles and Archangel Jophiel—the angel of inner wisdom and beauty—to aid in a romantic relationship. This oil also invites assistance from Kuan Yin, goddess of mercy, and Mother Mary as the Divine Mothers of wisdom and compassion. Use jasmine to help you connect to your beloved. This oil assists in bringing in good memories and the pure teachings of Atlantis.

Mental uses Use jasmine to renew your self-confidence and increase your courage to put good thoughts into action. It also supports you as you lighten up and allow yourself to feel good about yourself. In cases of depression, jasmine is a helpful addition to other steps taken; it has been known to be helpful in cases of severe depression, but it is not a substitute for other remedies.

Emotional uses Jasmine increases the courage you need to embrace the magnificent person you truly are. It is also advantageous when you are trying to absorb all that is going on in your life and the lives of those around you. Jasmine is said to activate endorphins, bringing about feelings of well-being and euphoria.

Physical uses Use jasmine in synergistic blends to improve sexual desire, increase sperm count, and alleviate impotence. This oil is beneficial to help calm nerves and promote sound sleep. It balances hormones and eases the birthing and recovery process. It shortens the post-natal period and combats postpartum depression. Jasmine increases milk secretion. Jasmine is useful for pain relief and is often used in anti-aging skin products for its ability to help fade scars, marks, and wrinkles. It is also helpful for releasing addictions. Jasmine is a good aromatherapy ally for angel communicators, doulas, drug-rehabilitation specialists, fertility specialists, grief counselors, gynecologists, marriage counselors, maternity nurses, mental health counselors, mystics, and sex therapists.

Therapeutic properties Analgesic, antibacterial, antidepressant, antifungal, anti-inflammatory, antipruritic, antiseptic, antispasmodic, antistress, antitussive, antiviral, aphrodisiac, calmative, carminative, cicatrizant, decongestant, emollient, euphoriant, galactagogic, germicidal, parturient, sedative, stimulative (uterine contractions), tonic (female reproductive system), uplifting.

Divine guidance Do you need more sweetness in your life? Are you gentle with yourself? Treat yourself with kindness. Are you ready for a romantic relationship? Do you joyously give but find it difficult to receive? It is safe to allow others to do nice things for you and to shower you with gifts. Permit blessings and love to pour into your open, receptive heart. It's time to receive with grace.

For your safety Pregnant women should avoid using jasmine before they are at the actual birth process because it is an emmenagogue (an agent that promotes menstrual discharge). It is highly relaxing and sedating; therefore, avoid heavy doses of jasmine.

Interesting tidbits:

Jasmine has been used since ancient times in rituals, ceremonies, baths, and teas. The flower has been used as an adornment for hair. This florally scented oil has founds its way into many popular fragrances, including Patou's *Joy*, Yves Saint Laurent's *Rive Gauche,* and Dior's *Diorella.*

JUNIPER BERRY
Detoxification

BOTANICAL NAME	*Juniperus communis*
NOTE	middle
METHOD OF EXTRACTION	steam distillation
PARTS USED	ripe berries
FRAGRANCE	fresh, resinous, woody
COLOR(S)	green, white
CHAKRA(S)	crown, third eye, navel
ASTROLOGICAL SIGN(S)	Pisces, Libra
PLANET(S)	Jupiter, Neptune, Venus
NUMBER(S)	22/4, 33
ANIMAL(S)	peacock, phoenix
ELEMENT(S)	fire

Affirmation I fully appreciate my transformation. My emotions are balanced, and I enjoy this state of being. Events from my past positively affect my present and future. I embrace change. I recognize that change can usher in improved life situations. I am grateful for the balanced flow of energy within me.

Complementary flower essences Agrimony to overcome addiction to alcohol, drugs, or sugar. *Crab Apple* for self-acceptance and balancing of inner harmony. *Walnut* to help while healing from attachments and habits.

Complementary stones Chlorite, phantom quartz, jet, orbicular jasper, smoky quartz, tree agate, watermelon tourmaline.

About the plant Juniper is an evergreen bush that reaches a height of up to 6 feet. It has silvery-green needlelike leaves and bluish-green cones that produce berries.

Chemical components Pinene, sabinene, myrcene, germacrene, limonene, cadinene, terpinen, caryophyllene, elemene.

Spiritual uses Just as juniper berry can be used to cleanse and detoxify your body, the same is true for cleansing your aura, or energy field. Use this oil to purify the atmosphere and to support spiritual connection. Juniper berry is beneficial to ward off negativity and evil intent. The spiritual wisdom of the plant kingdom and the devic forces of the plants can be accessed by working with this essential oil.

Mental uses Use juniper to detox your mind of repetitive negative thought patterns. It is beneficial when you want to break ties to anything that is holding you back from living a happy and fulfilled life, which starts with your thoughts and where your focus is placed.

Emotional uses Juniper berry oil is a good addition to a synergistic blend to help you release stress and improve your ability to relax. Juniper berry improves your potential to deal with your feelings and emotional difficulties. Inhale this essential oil and visualize a restoration of inner harmony and self-confidence.

Physical uses Juniper berry removes toxins from the body, especially in the case of drug abuse, alcoholism, and smoking. Juniper berry is a diuretic and is helpful for cleansing of the urinary tract through inhalation and topical application with a carrier oil on the soles of your feet. It is also a digestive aid. Juniper berry is a good aromatherapy ally for conservationists, drug rehabilitation specialists, farmers, florists, gardeners, healthcare professionals, and landscape architects.

Therapeutic properties Abortifacient, analgesic, antifungal, anti-inflammatory, antilithic, antiparasitic, antirheumatic, antiscorbutic, anti-septic, antispasmodic, antitoxic, antitussive, aphrodisiac, astringent, blood purifier, carminative, cholagogic, cicatrizant, depurative, detoxifier, digestive, diuretic (strong), emmenagogic, germicidal, hemostatic, insecticidal, nervine, refreshing, rubefacient, sedative, stimulative (genitourinary tract), stomachic, sudorific, tonic, tonifying, vulnerary.

Divine guidance Are you aware of your thoughts? Let go of your repetitive patterns. Focus on where you are going and manifest your best life. Remember your ability to flex and bend in a storm. Accept the transformational power of growth. Remember your roots; yet always remember how much you can grow to reach great heights. It's time to rev up your self-acceptance and self-love.

For your safety Avoid use in cases of kidney disease. Do not use if pregnant or nursing.

> **Interesting tidbits:**
> A branch of juniper was traditionally hung on doors on the eve of May Day to ward off witchcraft. In Italy, it was burned on Christmas Eve to deflect the evil eye, or *malocchio*. During the Middle Ages, juniper berries were burned to ward off the plague. Juniper is the overriding flavor in gin.

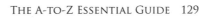

LAVENDER
Sweet Transformation

BOTANICAL NAME	*Lavandula officinalis*
NOTE	top to middle
METHOD OF EXTRACTION	steam distillation
PARTS USED	flowers
FRAGRANCE	clean, floral, fresh, green, herbaceous, light, mellow, sweet, warm, woody
COLOR(S)	green, lavender, purple, white
CHAKRA(S)	all
ASTROLOGICAL SIGN(S)	Aquarius, Virgo, Leo
PLANET(S)	Chiron, Earth, Moon, Sun
NUMBER(S)	11, 22, 33, 44
ANIMAL(S)	kitten, puppy
ELEMENT(S)	all

Affirmation I am healthy, whole, and complete. Peace and serenity are mine. I relax and breathe deeply, knowing all is well. I am grateful for sound sleep and pleasant dreams.

Complementary stones Amethyst, ametrine, angelite, apophyllite, celestite, charoite, clear quartz, chlorite quartz, green moss agate, hemimorphite, kambaba jasper, lapis lazuli, turquoise.

Complimentary Flower Essences *Cherry Plum* to feel calm and collected. *Red Chestnut* to stop worry and feel inner peace. *Rescue Remedy* to relieve sudden stress. *Star of Bethlehem* to release shock. *Vine* to quiet aggressiveness.

About the plant Lavender is an evergreen plant that is native to the Mediterranean, grows to a height of about 3 feet, and has light purple flowers.

Chemical components Linalyl acetate, linalool, coumarin, caryophyllene, geranyl acetate, terpinen, herniarin, farnesene, camphor, octen-3-yl acetate.

Spiritual uses Lavender is a great tool for meditation. This oil brings in blessings and the sweetness of love. Use this essential oil for channeling, trance mediumship, psychic development, and heightened spiritual awareness. The cleansing scent and vibe of this essential oil is ideal to deter jealousy and negative energies from others. The vibration of lavender aids in connecting with Archangel Sabrael, Saint Germain, and Kuan Yin, goddess of mercy and compassion. Add lavender oil to a mister filled with purified water to cleanse your yoga mat. The scent also aids your yoga practice. Add lavender to the water you use to clean your floors and countertops to remove negative energy and replace it with blessings and love. This essential oil assists in bringing back good memories and the pure teachings of Atlantis.

Mental uses The cleansing scent of lavender clears and calms the mind and brings about mental clarity, helping you to sort out the details and release chaos. It also relieves mental exhaustion, stress, and anxiety.

Emotional uses Lavender is comforting to your heart, soothing and calming chaotic and rampant emotions such as hysteria and worry. Lavender is an aid for dispelling the blues. Due to its relaxing and sedative nature, lavender is beneficial for challenging situations on all levels and for all ages. Inhale this essential oil while you repeat the affirmations above.

Physical uses The beneficial nature of lavender is so far-reaching that the list of its positive attributes could fill a book. If you could have only one essential oil in your cabinet, lavender would be the best oil to choose. Lavender's physical benefits include relief of aching muscles, improvement of acne, clearing infections, repelling insects, treating bacterial infections, healing burns and other minor wounds, soothing earaches, treating eczema, relieving fatigue, reducing fevers, relieving headaches, alleviating insomnia, easing menstrual cramps, balancing hormones in menopause, treating shingles, and relieving sinusitis. Lavender is a good aromatherapy ally for all walks of life.

Therapeutic properties Analgesic, antibacterial, antibiotic, anticonvulsive, antidepressant (premenstrual syndrome and menopause), antifungal, anti-inflammatory, antiparasitic, antirheumatic, antiseptic, antispasmodic, antistress, antitoxic, antitussive, antivenomous, antiviral, aperitive, calmative, carminative, cephalic, cholagogic, cicatrizant, cordial, cytophylactic, decongestant, deodorizer, detoxifier, diuretic, emmenagogic, healing (skin), hypotensor, insecticidal, nervine, regenerative (skin tissue), restorative, reviving, sedative (heart), stimulative (respiratory system), stomachic, sudorific, tonic, vulnerary.

Divine guidance Are you feeling a need for comfort? Do you want to be soothed or rocked to sleep by loving arms? Do you need to repel those pesky energies that are annoying and replace them with blessings? It is time to find the tools to bring you comfort. Take it into your own hands to do what it takes to make your life happier and filled with peace and calm.

For your safety No known contraindications.

Interesting tidbits:
Lavender gets its name from the Latin *lavare,* which means "to wash." Thieves who robbed victims of the plague during the Middle Ages actually used lavender as one of the ingredients in their vinegar-based concoction to protect them from becoming infected. (The other ingredients were garlic, rosemary, and thyme.) Although lavender is a lover of dry, sunny, and rocky habitats, English gardeners and gardeners of the Pacific Northwest are renowned for growing lavender plants. Lavender buds have been used as sachets to scent linens and clothing while deterring moths and insects.

LEMON
Brilliance

BOTANICAL NAME	*Citrus limon*
NOTE	top
METHOD OF EXTRACTION	cold-press
PARTS USED	fruit peel
FRAGRANCE	bright, clean, fresh
COLOR(S)	yellow
CHAKRA(S)	solar plexus
ASTROLOGICAL SIGN(S)	Taurus, Gemini, Leo
PLANET(S)	Mercury, Sun, Venus
NUMBER(S)	24/6
ANIMAL(S)	blue-and-gold macaw, fox, hummingbird, parakeet, sloth
ELEMENT(S)	air, fire

Affirmation I am confident and courageous. I shine my light brightly for all to see. I honor and respect myself for who I am and what I can do. I am blessed with mental clarity. It is easy for me to integrate all that is going on around me.

Complementary flower essences Cerato to trust your own inner knowing. *Gentian* to move forward even when faced with setbacks. *Larch* to release pessimism and perceived blocks. *Rock Rose* for confidence and to release panic.

Complementary stones Citrine, golden calcite, yellow topaz, yellow tourmaline, serpentine, lemon/citron chrysoprase, peridot, light-green jade.

About the plant Lemon is an evergreen citrus tree that grows to a height of about 10 to 20 feet with white flowers that develop into yellow fruit.

Chemical components Limonene, pinene, terpinene, terpineol, geranial, sabinene, cymene, myrcene, neral, terpinen, neryl acetate.

Spiritual uses Lemon connects you with your Divine nature, activating a blissful connection with the Divine. The more aware you are of this aspect of your spiritual body, the more you will actualize the benefits of the connection with higher consciousness.

Mental uses Lemon brings mental clarity, helping you to focus your attention on work, especially when dealing with important details. It helps you look at things from various angles for a greater perspective. Use lemon to assist you when you want to become conscious of the repetitive patterns of self-limiting thoughts that are holding you back. Then develop and focus on positive thoughts to replace those negative beliefs. Inhale this essential oil while you repeat the affirmations above.

Emotional uses Use lemon oil in synergistic blends to help raise your spirits. It assists you in garnering self-confidence when you are on a quest to improve your self-esteem. Lemon helps when you are recovering from the blues as it aids in releasing the symptoms of depression. The golden energy of this oil can help dissipate whatever challenge or negative emotion is blocking your way to happiness.

Physical uses The purifying nature of lemon cleanses and detoxifies. This oil is a great aid for weight loss and improved digestive function. Use lemon to restore vitality after a prolonged illness to release physical exhaustion and refresh the body on all levels. It is a tonic for the circulatory system and is good in a synergistic blend with oregano to ease pressure on varicose veins. Lemon is a good aromatherapy ally for accountants, bankers, lawyers, healthcare practitioners, housekeepers, infectious disease specialists, leaders, pilots, and any profession that requires thorough and unwavering focus.

Therapeutic properties Antianemic, antibacterial, antibiotic, antidepressant, antifungal, antilithic, antineuralgic, antioxidant, antiparasitic, antipruritic, antirheumatic, antisclerotic, antiscorbutic, antiseptic (strong), antispasmodic, antistress, antitoxic, antitussive, antiviral, aperitive, astringent, blood purifier, calmative, carminative, cephalic, cicatrizant, coagulant, cooling, decongestant, depurative, detoxifier, diaphoretic, digestive, disinfectant, diuretic, emollient, febrifugal, hemostatic, hepatic, hypotensor, insecticidal, invigorating (immune system), laxative, refreshing, rubefacient, sedative, stimulative (circulatory and lymphatic systems), stomachic, tonic, uplifting.

Divine guidance Are you trying to gain clarity? Do you embrace your personal power? Are you aware of your brilliance? Acknowledge your magnificence. You do have the ability to stay focused and alert. Focus on what you do well to increase your self-esteem. Trust that it is safe to be powerful in a loving way. Shine your light to reach your full potential!

For your safety This oil is phototoxic; therefore, avoid exposure to direct sunlight when using topically.

> ### Interesting tidbits:
> Ancient Egyptians used lemon on fish and meat to avoid food poisoning. Lemons were introduced to Europe by crusaders during the early Middle Ages. When the aroma of lemon essential oil is diffused into the air in office buildings, it is believed to improve worker focus and reduce error.

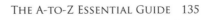

LEMONGRASS
Verve

BOTANICAL NAME	*Cymbopogon citratus*
NOTE	top
METHOD OF EXTRACTION	steam distillation
PARTS USED	leaves (fresh or partly dried)
FRAGRANCE	fresh, lemony, sweet, fruity, earthy
COLOR(S)	pale to vivid yellow
CHAKRA(S)	solar plexus, navel
ASTROLOGICAL SIGN(S)	Leo, Scorpio
PLANET(S)	Sun
NUMBER(S)	6
ANIMAL(S)	bee, hummingbird
ELEMENT(S)	fire

Affirmation I am grateful for the sense of belonging I have with friends, family, and colleagues. The blessings of self-confidence are with me daily. I am energized, and I have plenty of endurance. I am peaceful and healthy!

Complementary flower essences *Elm* for endurance and staying focused on the present moment. *Hornbeam* for feeling overwhelmed and lacking enthusiasm. *Oak* to relax if you are a relentless overachiever. *Olive* to give yourself time to rest and rejuvenate.

Complementary stones Carnelian, chrysoprase, citrine, yellow chrysoprase, sunstone.

About the plant Native to India and preferring full sun, lemongrass is a grassy plant with sword-like leaves that reaches a height of about 3–6 feet.

Chemical components Myrcene, citronellal, geranyl acetate, nerol, geraniol, neral (traces of limonene and citral).

Spiritual uses Lemongrass is useful for clearing the mind and your space prior to contemplation, meditation, and prayer. Use it to call upon Archangel Ariel, the angel of general health and vitality.

Mental uses Lemongrass invigorates and promotes clarity. It also increases joyfulness and enthusiasm while helping you to process all that is going on around you. Use it to improve your ability to see life with joy, to relieve stress, and to restore balance after a stressful period.

Emotional uses Lemongrass is useful to improve feelings of belonging, working in harmony with others, and compatibility. Improve your self-confidence through inhalation of this essential oil while matching it with the affirmation above.

Physical uses Use lemongrass to relieve achy joints, lower high blood pressure, and to kill germs. In a carrier oil, lemongrass massaged into the muscles improves their suppleness, increases circulation, and reduces muscle pain. This oil also alleviates excessive perspiration and helps to clear up acne and oily skin. It makes a good insect repellent, reduces pet odors, and generally deodorizes the air. It can be used for headache relief and even reduces the symptoms of jet lag. Lemongrass helps keep pets free of ticks and fleas. (Confirm with your veterinarian prior to use on your pet.) Lemongrass is a good aromatherapy ally for environmentalists and pest control professionals.

Therapeutic properties Analgesic, antibacterial, antidepressant, antifungal, antimicrobial, antiperspirant, antiseptic, antiviral, astringent, carminative, deodorizer, diuretic, febrifugal, galactagogic, insecticidal, nervine, sedative (nervous system), tonic.

Divine guidance Are you having a challenge integrating all that goes on around you? Is it hard to think clearly, finding your thoughts are congested? Allow the flow of the brilliant sunlight to bring clarity and energize your life with peace and calm.

For your safety Use in small amounts diluted to 1% or less for skin applications. Possible skin irritant. Do not use if pregnant or nursing.

> ### Interesting tidbits:
> Lemongrass, which works as an attractant pheromone, is used as a "swarm trap" to lure bees to a bait beehive. It is a culinary herb used in Asian cuisine. It has been used as a zesty tea for coughs and digestion. The plant in the yard is said to repel mosquitoes.

LIME
Clarity and Joy

BOTANICAL NAME	*Citrus aurantifolia*
NOTE	top
METHOD OF EXTRACTION	cold-press
PARTS USED	fruit peel
FRAGRANCE	citrusy, fresh, sweet
COLOR(S)	green
CHAKRA(S)	heart, solar plexus, third eye
ASTROLOGICAL SIGN(S)	Leo, Virgo
PLANET(S)	Sun
NUMBER(S)	22
ANIMAL(S)	coyote, fox, hummingbird
ELEMENT(S)	fire

Affirmation I have great mental clarity. I am alert and uplifted. I have boundless inner peace and joy. I feel grateful for my happiness and the sweetness of life!

Complementary flower essences Clematis for staying present and connected. *Gentian* to feel confident and embrace enthusiasm. *Larch* to release fears and perceived blocks and to recognize opportunities. *Mustard* to overcome depression and feel delight.

Complementary stones Clear quartz, citrine, green kyanite, peridot, light-green jade, yellow fluorite.

About the plant Native to Asia, lime is an evergreen that grows to a height of up to 10 feet with fragrant white flowers that develop into green fruit.

Chemical components Limonene, pinene, terpinene, sabinene, geranial, bisabolene, neral, myrcene, bergamotene, caryophyllene, farnesene.

Spiritual uses Lime helps you connect with higher spiritual guides and angels. The bright, happy scent of lime adds joy to a spiritual practice and uplifts your consciousness to invite higher thoughts. Lime is a good tool to use for periods of contemplation and integration.

Mental uses Lime brings mental clarity. Use it when you need to feel more alert. This oil is a good work or study aid and can be helpful for avoiding errors in detailed work. The sweet scent of lime helps to counteract dark thoughts and bring awareness to the sweetness of life.

Emotional uses Lime assists you in feeling joy and finding inner peace. Use it to recover from periods of the blues or low self-esteem. This oil raises your awareness so you can work through your feelings, validate them, and move on to more joyful pursuits. Place a bit of lime oil in a diffuser or on a hanky to inhale while journaling to achieve both emotional and mental clarity.

Physical uses Because of its antiseptic properties, lime in a carrier oil for topical use is beneficial for preventing and assisting in the healing of infections. Lime also helps to clear up respiratory infections and helps relieve bronchitis, coughs, and colds. Its cooling qualities help to reduce fevers. Due to its antiviral qualities, in a synergistic blend it can help heal and discourage a shingles outbreak. It is also known for its disinfecting abilities, so add it to a spray bottle with purified water and other disinfectant oils for cleaning the kitchen and bathroom. Lime is a good aromatherapy ally for accountants, bankers, caregivers, chefs, ear/nose/throat specialists, editors, manicurists, and mental health counselors.

Therapeutic properties Antibacterial, antidepressant, antilithic, antioxidant, antirheumatic, antisclerotic, antiscorbutic, antiseptic, antispasmodic, antitoxic, antiviral, aperitive, astringent, cooling, depurative, disinfectant, febrifugal, hemostatic, hepatic, insecticidal, refreshing, restorative, stimulative (digestive and lymphatic systems), tonic (immune system), uplifting.

Divine guidance Are you feeling a bit foggy and unclear? Do you find yourself a bit sleepy when you need to stay focused on details? Perhaps you are a bit insecure or feeling down because of the magnitude of work ahead? Inhale lime oil and make a clear intention that as you breathe deeply your mind is clear and alert. Remember your passion for life, living, and your work, and your day will refill itself with joy and clarity!

For your safety This oil is phototoxic; therefore, avoid exposure to direct sunlight when using topically.

> **Interesting tidbits:**
> Lime's high vitamin C content helped to prevent (and sometimes cure) scurvy among nineteenth-century English sailors. This is how the expression "limey" came about.

Mandarin
Sweet Peace and Comfort

BOTANICAL NAME	*Citrus reticulata*
NOTE	top
METHOD OF EXTRACTION	cold-press
PARTS USED	fruit peel
FRAGRANCE	citrusy, sweet, candy-like
COLOR(S)	orange, pink
CHAKRA(S)	heart, navel, solar plexus
ASTROLOGICAL SIGN(S)	Aries, Aquarius, Leo, Libra
PLANET(S)	Sun, Uranus, Venus
NUMBER(S)	7, 11, 22, 44, 52
ANIMAL(S)	dragon, dragonfly, fox, hummingbird, lizard
ELEMENT(S)	air, fire

Affirmation I have an abundance of spiritual helpers assisting me in all areas of my life. Guidance and inspiration from my angels and other spirit guides come to me moment by moment. I am blessed with nurturing vibrations wherever I go!

Complementary flower essences *Aspen* for undefined fears. *Clematis* for focus. *Mimulus* for courage. *Red Chestnut* for peace.

Complementary stones Angelite, celestite, carnelian, clear quartz, hematite, morganite, kunzite, orange calcite, pink calcite.

About the plant Native to China, mandarin is a citrus fruit tree that grows to a height of up to 25 feet tall.

Chemical components Limonene, terpinene, pinene, myrcene, cymene, thujene, terpinolene.

Spiritual uses Mandarin helps you to connect with your guardian angels, who act and react based on thoughtforms and specific requests. Because humans have free will, angels need to be asked to assist us or intervene on our behalf. As you inhale mandarin, imagine a clear connection with your guardian angel and ask for specific assistance and guidance. Mandarin oil aligns with inner peace, safety, and sweet dreams on a vibrational level. Use this oil to call upon Archangel Michael for intelligence, observation, and perspective; upon Archangel Gabriel for inspiration and guidance, dream interpretation, and inner knowing; and upon Archangel Auriel to realign with the Divine Feminine and to release your subconscious fears. This essential oil assists in bringing back good memories and the pure teachings of Atlantis.

Mental uses Mandarin is uplifting and adds positive energy to your thoughts. It helps you shift from a negative outlook to a positive one—the great transition from the half-empty glass to a *full* glass (notice that it is not just half-full). Like its citrus relatives, mandarin brings mental clarity and sharpens the mind.

Emotional uses Use mandarin in situations in which you need to elicit feelings of safety. It is especially helpful to add this sweet scent and energy to a synergistic blend for young children when they are feeling fearful at bedtime or are afraid of the dark. This oil has a calming effect and the vibration of sweet candy. Mandarin aids in encouraging pleasant dreams and releases the emotional stress resulting from nightmares.

Physical uses Mandarin promotes restful sleep because of its sedative properties. It strengthens the liver and facilitates digestion by stimulating the digestive juices. It can be used to increase the appetite. It improves circulation and relieves spasms. Mandarin is a good aromatherapy ally for angel communicators, bakers, children, entrepreneurs, Feng Shui practitioners, musicians, parents, and mental health counselors.

Therapeutic Properties Antidepressant, antiemetic, antiseptic, antispasmodic, antistress, antitussive, aperitive, astringent, calmative, carminative, cholagogic, cytophylactic, decongestant, depurative, digestive, diuretic, emollient, hypnotic, revitalizing, sedative, stimulant (digestive and lymphatic systems), stomachic, tonic, uplifting.

Divine guidance Are you ready to attract the best of everything? Do you believe the best is yet to come? Make a clear decision to manifest the good now, in this moment.

For your safety This oil is phototoxic; therefore, avoid exposure to direct sunlight when using topically.

> **Interesting tidbits:**
> Mandarin oranges, as well as clementines and tangerines, are symbols of abundance and good luck. They are often given as gifts during the Chinese New Year. In some homes, it is a traditional Christmas ritual to place mandarins or tangerines in the Christmas stockings.

MELISSA
You Catch More Bees with Honey

BOTANICAL NAME	*Melissa officinalis*
NOTE	middle
METHOD OF EXTRACTION	steam distillation
PARTS USED	leaves
FRAGRANCE	lemony, sweet
COLOR(S)	pastel blue, pink, white, yellow
CHAKRA(S)	root, navel, solar plexus
ASTROLOGICAL SIGN(S)	Taurus
PLANET(S)	Venus
NUMBER(S)	4
ANIMAL(S)	bee, butterfly, hawk, sloth
ELEMENT(S)	air, earth

Affirmation I am aligned with the healing powers of inner peace and kindness. I am able to help others by vibrating love through my presence, words, and actions. I am gentle with myself. I recognize that kindheartedness brings about better life situations.

Complementary flower essences Impatiens for a more re-laxed approach to life. *Oak* for exhaustion. *Vervain* to relieve tension and step into stillness. *Vine* to encourage kindness and compassion.

Complementary stones Amethyst, blue calcite, citrine, golden cal-cite, golden topaz, honey calcite, magenta-dyed agate, malachite.

About the plant Melissa is a perennial bushy herb in the mint family that reaches a height of up to 3 feet; it has serrated leaves and small white or pink flowers.

Chemical components Geranial, neral, caryophyllene, citronelial, germacrene, caryophyllene oxide, geranyl acetate, methyl-5-hepten-2-one, copaene, methyl citronellate, terpineol, caryophyllene, nerol, octen-3-ol.

Spiritual uses Melissa improves the ability to meditate and visualize. Imagination is the key to improving intuition and facilitating a deeper connection with the angelic realm and loved ones on the Other Side. This oil helps you to be open to receive messages and guidance while raising your confidence that you are not "making up" your intuitive experience. Use melissa as a dreamtime tool to receive dreams for healing and prophecy.

Mental uses Melissa is helpful for rebalancing the mind due to the loss of mental functions, such as thinking, memory, and reasoning. It has been used for dementia, not the disease itself, but rather a group of symptoms caused by various health conditions. It is beneficial for relaxing and releasing the agitation associated with dementia, Alzheimer's disease, and sundown syndrome.

Emotional uses Melissa has a calming effect, so it is useful in cases of anxiety as well as ADD/ADHD. Melissa calms raging emotions in general. Because of its stress-relieving qualities, it may help to reduce high blood pressure. Use melissa to uplift your spirits and chase away the blues; it also helps relieve of the symptoms of depression.

Physical uses Melissa helps to heal wounds and suppress inflammation. Add melissa to a synergistic blend along with bergamot, eucalyptus radiata, geranium, lavender, and ravensara for relief of pain and healing of a shingles outbreak. I've provided many a family member and friends with this combination and they indicated they have had amazing results. Add this synergistic blend to coconut oil and rub it onto the soles of your feet before bed and before you start your day. Melissa is great as a sleep aid. It improves digestion and helps to relieve flatulence, upset stomach, and bloating. Use it for relief from menstrual cramps and general aches. Melissa is a good aromatherapy ally for angel communicators, beekeepers, caregivers, conservationists, and hospice caregivers.

Therapeutic properties Analgesic, antibacterial, antibiotic, anticonvulsive, antidepressant, anti-inflammatory, antioxidant, antiparasitic, antiputrid, antiseptic, antispasmodic, antistress, antiviral, aperitive, calmative, carminative, cephalic, choleretic, cytophylactic, diaphoretic, digestive, emmenagogic, febrifugal, galactagogic, hypotensor, insecticidal, nervine, sedative, stomachic, tonic, uplifting, vulnerary.

Divine guidance Are you using up your time being busy? Are you a workaholic? Or are you busy enough? Find a balance of relaxation and productivity. Take time to smell the sweetness of life around you. Remember that your life's activities are more productive and enjoyable when you take time to appreciate them.

For your safety Possible skin irritant. Do not use if pregnant or nursing.

> *Interesting tidbits:*
> Melissa is also known as balm or balm mint. The Swiss-German Renaissance physician Paracelsus referred to melissa as the "elixir of life." This herb was among those used during the Middle Ages on the floors of homes for their ability to mask or remove foul odors, for their insecticidal and antiseptic qualities, and to repel evil. Herbs used for this purpose were called "strewing herbs."

Myrrh
Stabilize and Preserve

BOTANICAL NAME	*Commiphora myrrha*
NOTE	base
METHOD OF EXTRACTION	steam distillation
PARTS USED	bark
FRAGRANCE	dark, opulent, mushroom-like, resinous, rich, warm, woody; reminiscent of wet wood
COLOR(S)	brown, black, gray, white
CHAKRA(S)	crown, root
ASTROLOGICAL SIGN(S)	Cancer, Libra
PLANET(S)	Moon, Venus
NUMBER(S)	17/8
ANIMAL(S)	camel, dog
ELEMENT(S)	air, water

Affirmation I am Divinely protected. All is well, and life is good. If I become distracted, I easily refocus my efforts. I honor my grounded connection with Mother Earth. I align my consciousness with gentleness, compassion, and goodwill toward all. My focus is on compassion and kindness.

Complementary flower essences *Heather* to stay focused and present in connection with others. *Star of Bethlehem* to realign after a death or traumatic experience. *Walnut* to balance emotions during times of change. *White Chestnut* to help you sleep and eliminate repetitive thoughts.

Complementary stones Ammonite, black tourmaline, brown agate, green calcite, honey calcite, Isis crystal, clear quartz, smoky quartz.

About the plant Myrrh is a tree native to Africa and Asia that grows to an average height of 12 feet; it can also be a small, thorny shrub that grows on rocky terrain.

Chemical components Furanoeudesma, furanodiene, lindestrene, elemene, germacrene, methoxyfuranodiene, isofuranogermacrene, cadinol, caryophyllene, bourbonene, cadinene.

Spiritual uses Myrrh is especially beneficial for grounding. Use it for protection in spiritual ceremonies and rituals. Considered a biblical oil, myrrh assists you in aligning with Christ Consciousness, as well as with the wisdom of Mother Mary, Mary Magdalene (the feminine Christ), Isis (goddess of transformation and life), and the archangels. High priests use it as an anointing oil. This oil is useful to fumigate or clear out negativity.

Mental uses Use myrrh to stabilize your thoughts and fix your attention on the vibration of safety. It helps you go within to uncover truths with an even keel. It helps you resolve problems when thoughts are spiraling and need to be grounded so that you can make sense of it all. Myrrh helps eliminate doubt and worry when you are faced with chaos and/or confusion. This oil helps you feel safe and sound.

Emotional uses Myrrh helps to heal, stabilize, and sedate rampant emotions, and cauterize energetic wounds from trauma. Combine with smoky quartz, frankincense, and lavender in a synergistic blend to calm you on an energetic level after a trauma. Use myrrh to bring your challenges into the light, observe them, and allow the light to transform and transmute stuck emotions and feelings that hold you back from achieving your full potential.

Physical uses Myrrh is a physical relaxant. It is useful in a synergistic blend to calm you for a sound sleep. Myrrh is a fixative and stabilizes the fragrance of a synergistic blend. According to Jennifer Peace Rhind's book *Fragrance and Wellbeing*, myrrh is helpful for healing wounds and sores on the gums and mouth as well. It soothes inflamed tissue. It has traditionally been used to lower blood sugar levels. Myrrh is a good aromatherapy ally for caregivers, dental professionals, judges, law enforcement professionals, lawyers, hospice workers, those who assist the dying to pass from this reality to the next, mediums, and others who communicate with the dearly departed.

Therapeutic properties Analgesic, antidiabetic, antifungal, anti-inflammatory, antiputrid, antiseptic (strong) (infected gums), antispasmodic, antitussive, aperitive, astringent, carminative, cicatrizant, cooling, deodorizer, depurative, diuretic, drying, emmenagogic, fixative, hemostatic, hypoglycemient, invigorating (immune system), rejuvenative (skin cells), revitalizing (skin), sedative, stimulative (digestive system), stomachic, sudorific, tonic (stomach), tonifying (cleanses and tightens the skin), vulnerary.

Divine guidance Do you feel that you've been scattered lately? Are you feeling confused? Find your connection and ground yourself. Stay focused on what is important in your life. Establish a circle of protection to keep you on course. Do you hear dead people or are you ready to assist someone who is crossing over to be birthed into the next reality?

For your safety Potentially toxic in high concentrations, so use sparingly. Do not use if pregnant or nursing.

> *Interesting tidbits:*
> Ancient Egyptians used myrrh along with cinnamon, cedarwood, and other resins in the embalming process. Biblical literature states that, prior to his crucifixion, Jesus the Christ was offered myrrh mixed with wine (as a stupefying potion) to somewhat ease his ordeal.

NEROLI
Joy in the Present Moment

BOTANICAL NAME	*Citrus aurantium*
NOTE	top to middle
METHOD OF EXTRACTION	steam distillation
PARTS USED	flowers
FRAGRANCE	exotic, sweet, floral, metallic
COLOR(S)	coral, pink, peach, white
CHAKRA(S)	crown, heart
ASTROLOGICAL SIGN(S)	Libra, Scorpio
PLANET(S)	Juno, Moon, Pluto, Venus
NUMBER(S)	7, 11
ANIMAL(S)	peacock, white buffalo
ELEMENT(S)	water

Affirmation I am magnificent in every way. I have the strength to do anything I set out to do with loving intentions. I am gentle with myself. I enjoy loving relationships. I am blessed with nurturing vibrations wherever I go.

Complementary flower essences Chestnut Bud to bring awareness and release the pattern of repetitive mistakes. *Elm* to improve self-confidence. *Oak* for self-nurturing. *Walnut* to adjust to the natural changes and cycles of life.

Complementary stones Angelite, blue lace agate, clear quartz, cobaltoan calcite, girasol quartz, kunzite, moonstone, pink calcite, rhodochrosite, rose quartz, selenite.

About the plant *Citrus aurantium* is a bitter orange tree native to Italy that grows to a height of up to 30 feet.

Chemical components Linalool, limonene, linalyl acetate, ocimene, terpineol, pinene, geranyl acetate, nerolidol, geraniol, farnesol, neryl acetate, myrcene, sabinene, nerol, ocimene.

Spiritual uses Neroli aligns with all Ascended Masters and angels. It helps ensure that you align with the highest vibrations prior to channeling, mediumship, or any type of spiritual work. Use neroli oil to call upon Archangel Auriel to assist in the connection with the Divine Feminine and to release subconscious fears; upon Archangel Muriel for help rebalancing your emotions; and upon Archangel Jophiel to help you see and know your own beauty. Use it also to request assistance from Kuan Yin (goddess of mercy and compassion) and Mother Mary to help you feel nurtured and safe. This essential oil assists in bringing back good memories and the pure teachings of Atlantis.

Mental uses Neroli gently and quietly elicits courage and mental strength during challenging times. It aids in bringing about inner peace and calm for a quiet mind. According to Wanda Sellar's *The Directory of Essential Oils*, neroli is "soothing in highly emotional states, hysteria, and shock."

Emotional uses Neroli helps you overcome verbal, mental, and emotional abuse by jogging your memory to say a positive affirmation anytime old negative thoughts arise. Neroli helps you remember your perfect magnificence. It is especially helpful for rebalancing wayward emotions associated with perimenopause and menopause. Neroli can help during times of grief regardless of what you are grieving—a relationship, a loved one's passing, the way things used to be, your younger self, and beyond.

Physical uses Neroli is a woman's best friend to relieve discomfort associated with the menstrual cycle. Neroli's relaxing components aid as a muscle relaxant. It works well for calming overly energized children. It is useful in a synergistic blend to relieve stress by day and calm oneself for a sound sleep by night. This sweet scent is an aphrodisiac and is also a good aid for improving fertility due to its relaxing effects and ability to enhance sexual response. Neroli is a good aromatherapy ally for fertility specialists, gynecologists, mothers, musicians, mystics, and parents.

Therapeutic properties Analgesic, antibacterial, antidepressant, antifungal, antiseptic, antispasmodic, antistress, antiviral, aphrodisiac, astringent, blood purifier, calmative, carminative, cicatrizant, cordial, cytophylactic, deodorizer, digestive, emollient, euphoriant, hypnotic, hypotensor, regenerative (skin cells), sedative, tonic, uplifting.

Divine guidance Do you realize that you are magnificent? Believe in your magnificence and embrace your power. Do you need more sweetness in your life? Are you gentle with yourself in your words and thoughts? Treat yourself with kindness. Be your own best friend, and be the best friend you can be to others. Love and accept your emotional nature.

For your safety No known contraindications.

> ### Interesting tidbits:
> The tree was named for the sixteenth-century Italian princess of Nerola, who fragranced her clothing and writing materials with the oil. The flowers are associated with matrimonial purity. It is used as an ingredient in eau de colognes. Commonly used by prostitutes in early century Europe, neroli thereby received its reputation for being an aphrodisiac.

NIAOULI
Restore and Remember Soul Contracts

BOTANICAL NAME	*Melaleuca quinquenervia, Melaleuca viridiflora*
NOTE	top to middle
METHOD OF EXTRACTION	steam distillation
PARTS USED	leaves
FRAGRANCE	camphoraceous, clear, disinfectant-like, herbaceous, medicinal, penetrating, strong
COLOR(S)	gold, green, orange, white, yellow
CHAKRA(S)	root, navel, solar plexus, throat
ASTROLOGICAL SIGN(S)	Virgo, Leo, Scorpio
PLANET(S)	Earth, Pluto, Sun
NUMBER(S)	0
ANIMAL(S)	alligator, frog, hawk
ELEMENT(S)	water

Affirmation I understand the factors controlling my life. I know I am the one in control. I have the power to shine like a star!

Complementary flower essences Crab Apple to relieve feelings of being contaminated or infected. *White Chestnut* for a clear mind. *Wild Oat* to help you remember your right livelihood or soul path.

Complementary stones Golden calcite, moldavite, septarian, vanadinite.

About the plant Niaouli is an Australian evergreen tree with yellow-green bottlebrush flowers and leathery leaves; it grows near water and ranges in height from 3 to 90 feet.

Chemical components Viridiflorol, cineole, nerolidol, ledol.

Spiritual uses Niaouli's vibration catapults you to an awareness of your soul's purpose. The energy of this oil clears away the cobwebs of your consciousness to help you wake up and realize that the web is actually an interconnected network leading you inward to realize your soul agreements for this lifetime. With this oil, call upon your ancestors, master guides, and guardian angels for help downloading ideas and instructions to better traverse your earth path during this lifetime.

Mental uses Niaouli clears the mind and aids with focus and concentration. It can also help shift overly compulsive thoughts surrounding cleanliness and order. The energetic vibration of this oil can help you deal with life's more pressing issues while reassuring the part of your mind that uses up time on compulsive behaviors. Niaouli's aroma adds good energy to gaining clarity on your life's purpose. Use very small amounts—a whiff now and then—to help you visualize, imagine, and remind you that you are clear on your life path. It breaks down old repetitive thought patterns and reconstitutes them with a new flair.

Emotional uses The cleansing properties of this oil can be used to clear out negative emotions, specifically those that have been created during prolonged illness or long recuperation periods. The energetics of niaouli increases emotional strength so that feelings of being ill can reverse to help you retrace your way back to full vital health and well-being. Use niaouli for the disintegration of emotional states that have been firmly established in the navel and root chakras. Instead of total disintegration, niaouli destabilizes the negativity associated with the challenging memories or experiences. Therefore, this oil helps you reintegrate the lessons captured from the experience, making you a much more powerful person because of it.

for circulation and relieving pain caused by phlebitis or varicose veins, as well as for relieving muscular tension and aches. Oregano clears candida infection and intestinal worms and parasites from the intestinal tract. It is also effective for irritable bowels. Oregano is a diuretic. Just as it improves the energetics of the mind and the emotions, oregano improves physical vitality and endurance.

OREGANO
Vitality

BOTANICAL NAME	*Origanum vulgare*
NOTE	middle to top
METHOD OF EXTRACTION	steam distillation

About the plant Palmarosa is a fragrant grass that reaches heights of up to 9 feet. It has red flowers.

Chemical components Geraniol, geranyl acetate, farnesol, linalool, ocimene, caryophyllene, geranial, caryophyllene oxide, myrcene, elemol, farnesol.

Spiritual uses Palmarosa clears your auric field when you need to energetically clear and calm your energetic space. It is useful in your meditation practice for expanding your sphere of love. Use this oil to invoke the assistance of Archangels Chamuel, Gabriel, Haniel, and Metatron for communication, guidance, and alignment with soul purpose.

Mental uses Palmarosa is useful for decompressing and releasing pressure in your mind. It helps to expand your mental pathways so that you can more easily generate new ideas. It helps you activate the basic fuel for your mind to ignite creative thoughts and provide solutions outside the norm.

Emotional uses Palmarosa is helpful for reducing stress and anxiety. Use it as an aid when you are trying to release problems and truly want to let them go. This oil can help release any anxiety you are feeling and allow your affairs to unfold with ease. Add this scent to synergistic blends to help let go of feelings of insecurity/lack of confidence and to help drive away the blues and relieve the symptoms of depression. Palmarosa adds a positive vibration to your energy field, resulting in balance.

Physical uses Palmarosa is perfect to add to a synergistic blend for premenstrual syndrome and hormonal imbalances. It is a pleasant alternative for fighting fungal infections like athlete's foot. It helps with stress-related challenges and heals frayed nerves. It has been known to aid in rebalancing digestion and intestinal flora. It acts as a catalyst for the appetite and has been known to help those suffering from anorexia. Palmarosa is a good aromatherapy ally for counselors, gastroenterologists, life coaches, meditation facilitators/practitioners, mental health counselors, and neurologists.

Therapeutic properties Abortifacient, analgesic, antibacterial, antifungal, antiparasitic, antiseptic, antispasmodic, antistress, antiviral, aperitive, aphrodisiac, astringent, calmative, carminative, cicatrizant, cytophylactic, digestive, emmenagogic, emollient, febrifugal, nervine, refreshing, regenerative (skin cells), sedative, sudorific, stimulative (circulatory and digestive systems), tonic, uplifting.

Divine guidance Do you need to gain perspective on your feelings? Are you allowing the tears to flow when the emotion arises? It is always good to look at things from different perspectives. Go with the flow and find a unique way to perceive your reality.

For your safety No known contraindications.

Interesting tidbits:
Palmarosa is sometimes called Indian geranium oil or gingergrass. Palmarosa is from the same family as lemongrass and citronella.

PALO SANTO
Sacred Wood

BOTANICAL NAME	*Bursera graveolens*
NOTE	top to middle
METHOD OF EXTRACTION	steam distillation
PARTS USED	dead branches and wood
FRAGRANCE	fresh, minty, musky, resinous, very strong, woody
COLOR(S)	brown, black, gray, metallic red
CHAKRA(S)	all
ASTROLOGICAL SIGN(S)	Scorpio
PLANET(S)	Pluto
NUMBER(S)	5
ANIMAL(S)	crow, dog, lizard
ELEMENT(S)	air, earth

Affirmation I am mindful of the energetic connections between others and myself. I automatically remove unhealthy cords of attachment that affect me mentally, emotionally, physically, and spiritually. I am grounded and focused.

Complementary flower essences Aspen for fear of the unknown. *Chicory* to release worry about safety of friends and family. *Mimulus* to overcome known fears. *Rescue Remedy* for overcoming everyday fears.

Complementary stones Black obsidian, black tourmaline, hematite, jet.

About the plant Native to Mexico, Peru, Ecuador, and Venezuela, palo santo is a tree that grows to a height of up to 60 feet tall with gray bark, green leaves, and small flowers.

Chemical components Limonene, menthofuran, terpineol, carvone, germacrene, pulegone, muurolene, carveol.

Spiritual uses Palo santo is well-loved in shamanic circles. It purifies the energy of a sacred circle or ceremonial practice while invoking the energy of the ancestors to join forces with the shamanic practitioner. Use palo santo alongside sage and cedar in spiritual practice and meditation. Use to invoke the aid of Archangel Sabrael to release jealousy and negative forces. This oil helps you align with elders and medicine men, both living and in spirit, from indigenous cultures, especially from South American heritage. Palo santo is used to clear bad or negative energy and deflect psychic attack (negative energy sent from others.) Use this oil to bring clarity of the source of negative energy. It is beneficial during shamanic journeywork and can be used like an amulet of protection and to help reveal deeper spiritual truths.

Mental uses Palo santo helps you return to center when you feel out of balance. It helps you focus and set aside fears and distractions so that you can continue to achieve your goals. This oil clears negative mental energy associated with jealousy, negative self-talk, confusing mental chatter, and general chaos.

Emotional uses Palo santo helps to draw out dark, negative emotions so that they can be released. Use this oil in a synergistic blend with sage, cedar, lavender, and sweet marjoram when you overreact to a situation or a person and need to understand the reason for your negative reaction. Allow the aroma and the energetic components of this oil to help you locate the source of the emotional problem so you can begin to heal. Palo santo reduces anxiety and stress and uplifts your mood.

Physical uses Use palo santo, which eases congestion, to help clear your breathing passages. Add palo santo to pain-relieving and inflammation-reducing blends. It is calming to the immune system and is helpful as a restorative after an illness or stress. It helps to relieve pain and inflammation. This oil can also be used as a mosquito repellent. Palo santo is a good aromatherapy ally for Feng Shui practitioners, ghost hunters, intuitive readers, and shamanic practitioners.

Therapeutic properties Analgesic, anti-inflammatory, antimicrobial, diuretic, insecticidal.

Divine guidance Do you need to release the energetic cords attached to your ancestors and your past? Do you still have buttons that get pushed when you think of them? Take the time to recognize the patterns you are repeating from your parents and other family members established by your upbringing. Once you identify the belief systems and habits that were installed at a young age, then you can release those ties to your past. Unhook the mechanisms that push your buttons.

For your safety Do not use if pregnant or nursing.

> **Interesting tidbits:**
> Palo santo is endangered in Peru and threatened in Ecuador. Palo santo is also known as holy wood. It is in the same family as frankincense, myrrh, and elemi. I first encountered palo santo while apprenticing with a Peruvian spiritual teacher who burned it in circle teachings at the start of every session.

PATCHOULI
Love and Money

Botanical name	*Pogostemon cablin*
Note	base
Method of extraction	steam distillation
Parts used	leaves
Fragrance	earthy, sexy, sweet, hippy, musky, mossy, wine-like
Color(s)	amber, brown, green, yellow
Chakra(s)	heart, root, solar plexus
Astrological sign(s)	Aquarius, Pisces
Planet(s)	Uranus
Number(s)	1, 2, 11
Animal(s)	peacock, gorilla
Element(s)	air, water

Affirmation My energy abounds! I'm self-motivated to be productive. My tasks and creative projects are completed with ease. I am a caretaker of the earth and I take the time to enjoy nature. My connection with the fairies is strong. I intimately know and trust my inner truth. I meditate regularly.

Complementary flower essences Clematis for focus and grounding. *Hornbeam* for self-motivation. *Walnut* to stay grounded, even in the case of constant change.

Complementary stones Brown agate, green moss agate, green tourmaline, kambaba jasper, tree agate, ruby.

About the plant Patchouli is a large, bushy, hairy herb that reaches heights of about 3 feet with light purple flowers and oblong leaves.

Chemical components Bulnesene, guaiene, seychellene, patchoulene, caryophyllene, aromadendrene, pogostol, cadinene.

Spiritual uses Patchouli assists you in raising your consciousness to be more aware and present in the moment. Use it in spiritual practices to evoke sudden flashes of enlightenment or awakening of consciousness. It helps you to tap into the spiritual wisdom of the keepers, or devic forces, of the plant kingdom. Use it in shamanic practices to open a portal through which you can access the world of fairies, gnomes, and elves. Add a drop of patchouli to an aroma-energetic mist for mindful motion in your yoga practice.

Mental uses The earthy scent of patchouli is grounding. It brings focus and promotes action, thereby releasing laziness. Patchouli's aroma increases your awareness of issues or challenges, allowing you to perceive them from a higher perspective and thereby increasing your objectivity and ability to see the bigger picture.

Emotional uses Patchouli is uplifting and can assist you in shifting from a state of sadness to one of joy. Use it in synergistic blends with other uplifting oils, such as bergamot, lemon, and rosewood to raise self-confidence and self-worth. Patchouli can also help you to feel emotionally safe as it strengthens your sense of self.

Physical uses Patchouli is useful for repelling fleas, lice, and mosquitoes, especially in combination with eucalyptus radiata. It has been used for snakebites and is a good insect repellent. It also reduces and inhibits the growth of multiple strains of bacteria and fungi. Patchouli attracts both love and money. It works well in a synergistic blend as a fixative to stabilize the fragrance. Patchouli is a good aromatherapy ally for arborists, gardeners, landscape architects, neurologists, sex therapists, and yoga practitioners/instructors.

Therapeutic properties Alterative, analgesic, antibacterial, antibiotic, antidepressant, antiemetic, antifungal, anti-inflammatory, antiparasitic, antiphlogistic, antiseptic, antistress, antitoxic, antiviral, aphrodisiac, astringent (strong), calmative, carminative, cicatrizant (strong), cytophylactic, decongestant, deodorizer, diaphoretic, digestive, diuretic, febrifugal, fixative, insecticidal, laxative, nervine, regenerative (skin tissue), sedative (large amounts), stimulative (small amounts) (nerves), stomachic, tonic (uterus).

Divine guidance Do you wish to gain clearer insight or a better understanding of a situation? Make an appointment with yourself to meditate or sit in silence. Do this often. Open your consciousness and listen for your soul's truth and embrace it without judgment.

For your safety Has a stimulant effect when used excessively and a sedative effect when used sparingly.

> **Interesting tidbits:**
> Patchouli is used to scent India ink.

Pepper, Black
Take Action

BOTANICAL NAME	*Piper nigrum*
NOTE	top
METHOD OF EXTRACTION	steam distillation
PARTS USED	berries prior to ripening
FRAGRANCE	fresh, dry, masculine, warm, spicy, peppery, sometimes clove-like
COLOR(S)	black, gold, red, white
CHAKRA(S)	crown, third eye, root
ASTROLOGICAL SIGN(S)	Aries
PLANET(S)	Mars
NUMBER(S)	17/8, 27
ANIMAL(S)	antelope, dolphin, fox
ELEMENT(S)	air

Affirmation I am clear and focused mentally. I visualize my goals and aspirations effortlessly. I am self-assured. I step forward in life with confidence and purpose. I am grateful that my vital life force provides me with the energy and motivation to live life to the fullest!

Complementary flower essences *Gentian* to transform a negative attitude to one of positivity and enthusiasm. *Olive* for mental stress and exhaustion. *Sweet Chestnut* to improve endurance and strength. *Wild Oat* to improve mental processes regarding career and life path.

Complementary stones Channeling clear quartz, heliodor, Herkimer diamonds, kyanite, pietersite, rutilated quartz, selenite, tabular quartz.

About the plant Black pepper is a tropical vine native to India that grows to a height of 10 feet tall, with heart-shaped dark-green leaves and spiked white flowers that turn into berries.

Chemical components Caryophyllene, limonene, pinene, carene, sabinene, bisabolene, copaene, farnesene, cubebene.

Spiritual uses Black pepper activates the third eye. It is beneficial to help you open your mind to the spiritual realm and connect with spiritual teachers. Use black pepper in synergistic blends intended to develop your intuitive skills. This is a good oil to use to enhance the sensory gift of clairvoyance or psychic sight. Black pepper encourages your belief in your own inner knowing (clair-cognizance), and to take action on visions (clairvoyance) and the voice within (clairaudience). Call on Archangel Raziel while inhaling this essential oil to help you embrace your gifts of intuition and prophecy. This essential oil assists in bringing back good memories and the pure teachings of Atlantis.

Mental uses Black pepper stimulates your mind to speed up your thought processes and relieve sluggishness. Use black pepper to enhance memory and mental clarity. Use it as a main ingredient in a synergistic blend to help with mental acuity regarding business transactions.

Emotional uses Black pepper encourages emotional strength and endurance during challenging and sensitive times. The fiery vibration of black pepper helps burn away negative emotions by shining a bright light into the darkness. Use this oil to improve your personal self-worth and increase your self-esteem.

Physical uses Black pepper promotes energy and physical endurance. It is helpful to reduce fevers and stop bleeding. Add to a synergistic blend with celery seed oil and other analgesic oils to treat the pain of rheumatism and gout. Black pepper is an aromatherapy ally for actors, artists, graphic designers, musicians, writers, and any creative professional for tapping into the inspiration of doing their best, as well as environmentalists, mystics, and pest control professionals.

Therapeutic properties Analgesic, antibacterial, anticholinergic, anticonvulsive, antidote, antiemetic, antiseptic, antispasmodic, antitoxic, antitussive, aperitive, aphrodisiac, cardiac, carminative, detoxifier, diaphoretic, digestive, diuretic, febrifugal, insecticidal, laxative, rubefacient, sedative, stimulative (circulation; kidneys), stomachic, tonic, tonifying (muscles), vasodilator.

Divine guidance Do you desire more clarity and mental acuity? Become consciously aware of your thoughts with the help of this oil. You can discard the outdated thoughts and replace them with thoughts that focus on the life you want to live.

For your safety Possible skin irritant (low to moderate).

Interesting tidbits:
Pepper is one of the oldest known spices. It was used in India over 4,000 years ago to treat urinary infections and liver ailments. Greeks used it to alleviate fevers, and Romans used it to pay their taxes. In Rhind's *Fragrance and Wellbeing*, she states that black pepper, along with coriander, provides the spicy note to Dior's perfume *Miss Dior*.

PEPPERMINT
River of Creativity

BOTANICAL NAME	*Mentha piperita*
NOTE	top
METHOD OF EXTRACTION	steam distillation
PARTS USED	leaves and flowers
FRAGRANCE	clean, fresh, green, minty, overwhelming, strong
COLOR(S)	green, purple, white
CHAKRA(S)	all
ASTROLOGICAL SIGN(S)	Cancer, Pisces, Scorpio
PLANET(S)	Chiron, Mars, Moon, Pluto
NUMBER(S)	8
ANIMAL(S)	butterfly, fox, sloth, whale
ELEMENT(S)	water

Affirmation I glide through life with balance and grace. My mind is completely clear. My focused intent aligns me with my highest purpose. I use past experiences as valuable lessons, which allows me to propel forward in life with ease. I breathe deeply and know all is well.

Complementary flower essences Chestnut Bud to use lessons of the past to make good decisions in the future. *Rock Water* to integrate inner strength and to go with the flow. *Wild Oat* for clarity.

Complementary stones Apache tears, orbicular jasper, Orthoceras fossil, elestial crystal, time link quartz crystal.

About the plant Peppermint is a leafy green plant that reaches a height of 1 to 3 feet. It has fragrant leaves and violet flowers.

Chemical components Menthol, menthone, menthyl acetate, neo-menthol, cineole, menthofuran, isomenthone, pulegone, limonene, caryophyllene, sabinene hydrate.

Spiritual uses Peppermint can help you to remain truly present and awake during meditation. It is useful for regression therapy, rebirthing, or any practice that requires breathwork to maintain mindfulness to be truly present. Peppermint assists you in accessing past lives or earlier parts of this life, enabling you to heal and rebalance emotional and mental issues stemming from the past. Use peppermint to call on Archangel Muriel to help realign emotions.

Mental uses Peppermint helps to wake you up. Inhale this oil when you are experiencing mental fatigue. It's a great oil to have handy for long drives to maintain alertness. It stimulates mental clarity and focus. Peppermint holds the vibration of forward movement, propelling you ahead in the direction you need to go. While peppermint is helpful for digestion on a physical level, it also helps you digest life and truly understand and process all that is happening around and within you.

Emotional uses Peppermint can help you get in touch with your subconscious and the deep inner feelings you have for yourself and others. Use peppermint to sort out feelings. With peppermint nearby, take the time to journal and make a list of all that you are feeling so you can gain clarity and decide what you are ready to release. It also helps absorb and process what needs to be integrated to be able to move forward with enthusiasm. Peppermint is excellent to help drive away depressive thoughts and feelings.

Physical uses Peppermint relieves headaches and congestion. Use it as an aid to stay awake while driving. Peppermint relieves the itching and irritation of mosquito bites. Often used in foot lotion, it refreshes and relieves aching feet. Peppermint is especially helpful for digestion to relieve stomachaches and to activate digestive enzymes to detox the body. Peppermint is a good aromatherapy ally for dental professionals, environmentalists, neurologists, pest control professionals, pulmonary specialists, and regression therapists.

Therapeutic properties Alterative (mild), analgesic, anesthetic, antibacterial, antibiotic, anticonvulsive, antidepressant, antidiarrheal, antigalactagogic, anti-inflammatory, antineuralgic, antiparasitic, antiphlogistic, antipruritic, antiseptic, antispasmodic, antitoxic, antitussive, antiviral, aperitive, aphrodisiac, astringent, carminative, cephalic, cholagogic, cordial, decongestant, depurative, digestive, emmenagogic, febrifugal, hepatic, insecticidal, invigorating, nervine, refrigerant, restorative, stomachic, sudorific, tonic (heart), uplifting, vasoconstrictor.

Divine guidance Are you on the precipice of remembering your soul's purpose? Is it on the "tip of your tongue"? It is time to clear away your unhealthy repetitive patterns. Use your talents and focus instead on establishing peace and fellowship, starting with yourself, your family, your friends, and to extend your community. You have a special spiritual mission.

For your safety Possible skin irritant. Do not apply to sensitive areas, mucous membranes, or private parts. Keep away from eyes. Use in small quantities. May interfere with the efficacy of homeopathic remedies. Do not use if pregnant or nursing.

Interesting tidbits:

Cultivated in the thirteenth century, peppermint is actually a hybrid of spearmint and watermint. According to Greek mythology, the water nymph Mentha (aka Minthe), who had attracted the attention of Hades, was transformed into the mint plant as she was stomped on and beaten by the jealous goddess Persephone. Each blow released a delightful scent.

PETITGRAIN
Joyful Exuberance

BOTANICAL NAME	*Citrus aurantium*
NOTE	middle to top
METHOD OF EXTRACTION	steam distillation
PARTS USED	leaves, twigs, and young shoots
FRAGRANCE	citrusy, exotic, sweet, floral
COLOR(S)	green, orange, pink, white, yellow
CHAKRA(S)	heart, solar plexus
ASTROLOGICAL SIGN(S)	Leo, Sagittarius
PLANET(S)	Jupiter, Sun
NUMBER(S)	9
ANIMAL(S)	pelican
ELEMENT(S)	fire

Affirmation My light shines brightly. I am self-confident. Both others and I recognize my value and worth. I shine the light of compassion, kindness, and love from my heart.

Complementary flower essences Cerato for guidance and self-confidence. *Elm* to overcome feelings of depression. *Larch* for confidence. *Willow* to think positively.

Complementary stones Carnelian, citrine, clear quartz, golden calcite, green aventurine, rhodochrosite, rose quartz, selenite, sunstone.

About the plant *Citrus aurantium* is a bitter orange tree native to Italy that grows to a height of up to 30 feet.

Chemical components Linalyl acetate, linalool, terpineol, geranyl acetate, geraniol, neryl acetate, myrcene, ocimene, pinene, limonene.

Spiritual uses Petitgrain is a good go-to oil for uplifting, calming, and peaceful meditation experiences. Petitgrain helps you reduce the incessant chatter in your mind to allow for a positive meditation experience. This pleasant scent is a natural deodorizer, so it is beneficial in yoga classes and other types of workouts to balance the scents of perspiration. This essential oil assists in bringing back good memories and the pure teachings of Atlantis.

Mental uses Petitgrain shines light on mental obstacles. Use this oil for manifestation and to activate the power of the mind to create reality. This essential oil activates creative thought processes, helping you to bring forth inspiration. It calms the mind, relieves mental stress, supports mental activity, and increases positive thinking. Add this to a synergistic blend or use as a single note to activate good thoughts, a joyful outlook, and the ultimate in optimism.

Emotional uses Petitgrain is a calming aroma and therefore relieves agitated feelings. It is a perfect ingredient in synergistic blends for lifting you out of the blues and improving personal power and awareness.

Physical uses Petitgrain is a great oil to add to a peaceful-sleep blend. Due to its calming properties, it helps to ease breathing challenges and can be used to relieve muscle spasms. It also aids with digestion. Use petitgrain to clear up acne as well as isolated pimples. This is one of my favorite oils to add to synergistic blends for freshening and deodorizing the air. Petitgrain is a good aromatherapy ally for life coaches, massage therapists, meditation facilitators/practitioners, mental health counselors, musicians, neurologists, and veterinarians.

Therapeutic properties Antidepressant, antiseptic, antispasmodic, antistress, antiviral, astringent, calmative, deodorizer, digestive, fixative, nervine, refreshing, sedative, stimulative (digestive system), stomachic, tonic, uplifting.

Divine guidance Have you been feeling down in the dumps? Do you need to add some jazziness to your life? Do you need some brilliance and enthusiasm? This is a time of prosperity and purpose. You are ready to step into your power and be all that you were meant to be. You are aligned with the magnificence and the courage to show yourself in your fullest splendor!

For your safety No known contraindications.

> **Interesting tidbits:**
> Petitgrain translates to "little grains," which was originally derived from the fruit, not the leaves. This oil is often used in perfumery to lend an exotic scent to fragrances. Petitgrain is one of the ingredients in my oil blends created with the intention to improve self-confidence and relieve some of the symptoms of depression.

PINE
Mountain Air

BOTANICAL NAME	*Pinus sylvestris*
NOTE	middle
METHOD OF EXTRACTION	steam distillation
PARTS USED	needles and cones
FRAGRANCE	clean, coniferous, fresh, green, refreshing; reminiscent of the forest
COLOR(S)	brown, bluish green, green, red, turquoise
CHAKRA(S)	root
ASTROLOGICAL SIGN(S)	Capricorn, Sagittarius
PLANET(S)	Earth, Jupiter
NUMBER(S)	3
ANIMAL(S)	porcupine, turtle
ELEMENT(S)	air, earth

Affirmation I spend quality time in nature every day. I have an intimate connection with Mother Nature and her loving tools for natural healing. I find balance in all aspects of my life. The vibrant emerald-green energy of the plants and trees nurtures and restores my body, mind, and spirit.

Complementary flower essences Mimulus for oversensitivity. *Rock Rose* for strength and coping skills during challenging times. *Willow* to forgive and forget the past.

Complementary stones Black obsidian, green moss agate, howlite, red calcite, tree agate, turquoise.

About the plant Pine is a cone-producing evergreen tree that reaches heights of up to 130 feet. It has blue-green needle-like leaves.

Chemical components Borneol, bornyl acetate, terpinyl acetate, cadinene, camphene, dipentene, phellandrene, pinene, sylvestrene.

Spiritual uses Pine has a protective energy that benefits highly intuitive people. It helps to create a filter for, and barrier from, negative psychic energy and unwanted influences. Add pine to an aroma-energetic smudging mist for protection. Call on the ancestors with this essential oil in hand. This is a good oil for connecting with spiritual wisdom of the indigenous cultures. Inhale pine oil to amplify your understanding of the teachings of Native American spirituality or the way of the Good Red Road (walking the road of balance). Its energy lends itself to a stronger connection with Mother Earth and earth-centered spirituality. It is good for use in Sacred Circles and altars related to Native American ceremonies. Pine helps you align with the devic forces and nature spirits.

Mental uses Pine supports the mind during times of adverse conditions. It protects and strengthens the mind and prevents you from succumbing to the negativity that might arise around you in your home, office, or in any part of everyday life. The protective vibe of pine puts up a healthy barrier to prevent the telepathic receipt of others' negative thoughts.

Emotional uses Pine is helpful during times of potential emotional breakdown. It helps you release feelings of resentment, self-pity, and bitterness. Use pine if you are a highly sensitive person—like a sponge—for other people's feelings. It helps to protect you from absorbing the emotions of other people.

Physical uses Pine oil helps to cleanse the kidneys and clear up congested skin conditions like psoriasis and eczema. It helps to flush the lymphatic system and remove excess fluids from the body. Pine is antiseptic and offers relief from respiratory illness such as asthma, bronchitis, coughs, colds, and sinus infections. Use it to relieve pain, muscular exhaustion, and muscle aches as well as for relief from the symptoms of rheumatism. Pine oil encourages vitality and stimulates the adrenal glands. It's a great cleanser for the household. Pine oil is a good aromatherapy ally for arborists, conservationists, ecologists, infectious disease specialists, farmers, florists, gardeners, housekeepers, landscape architects, and law enforcement professionals.

Therapeutic properties Analgesic, antibacterial, antifungal, antineuralgic, antiparasitic, antiphlogistic, antirheumatic, antiscorbutic, antiseptic (strong), antispasmodic, antitussive, antiviral, cholagogic, choleretic, decongestant, deodorizer, depurative (kidneys), diuretic, hypertensor, insecticidal, laxative, refreshing, restorative, reviving, rubefacient, stimulative (circulatory and nervous systems; adrenal glands), sudorific, tonic, vulnerary.

Divine guidance Have you been feeling scattered lately and unable to focus on what's important? Look deeply inside, and you will see a reflection of all that is going on around you. Sort out what part of the reflection is really yours and what part really belongs to others. Prioritize your intentions, and focus on one thing at a time. Grounding yourself is important now so that you can accomplish your goals with sincerity and purpose. Consider exploring Native American spiritual teachings.

For your safety Possible skin irritant. Do not use if pregnant or nursing.

Interesting tidbits:
Ancient Egyptians used pine resin in the embalming process. Both Egyptians and Romans used pinecones as fertility charms. Pine nuts, also called *pignoli*, are a main ingredient in pesto sauce as well as in traditional Italian cookies.

 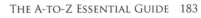

RAVENSARA
The Great Void, the Great Mystery

BOTANICAL NAME	*Ravensara aromatica*
NOTE	top
METHOD OF EXTRACTION	steam distillation
PARTS USED	leaves
FRAGRANCE	camphoraceous, herbaceous, woody
COLOR(S)	black, gold, green, shimmering metallic
CHAKRA(S)	crown, navel, root, throat
ASTROLOGICAL SIGN(S)	Libra, Scorpio
PLANET(S)	Pluto, Venus
NUMBER(S)	0, 5
ANIMAL(S)	bear, crow, owl, raven
ELEMENT(S)	fire

Affirmation I am focused and stay on track until a matter has reached a conclusion. I accomplish whatever I set out to do. I pay attention to what is going on around me and listen carefully to others as well as to myself. I am attentive to my own needs and to the needs of others.

Complementary flower essences Agrimony to help release emotional patterns and inner torment. *Chestnut Bud* to help you realize when or if you are making repetitive mistakes and to learn from your experiences. *White Chestnut* to release repetitive thoughts.

Complementary stones Black obsidian, golden sheen obsidian, tree agate, green moss agate.

About the plant Ravensara is a high-altitude tree that reaches heights of about 60 feet. It has aromatic leaves and bark.

Chemical components Limonene, sabinene, isoledene, estragole, caryophyllene, myrcene, terpinene, pinene, linalool, carene, terpinene, cineole, phellandrene, thujene, camphene, cadinene, copaene, cymene, elemene, ocimene.

Spiritual uses The vibration and aroma of ravensara draw you inward to the center of yourself. It brings you to the place of truth and wisdom. In Native American teachings, the energy associated with ravensara is likened to the Great Void or Great Mystery from which all things are created. Use ravensara to clear your consciousness and receive higher levels of prophetic dreaming or messages from a deeper part of yourself. Put your awareness on your navel chakra while using this oil to help you dream from the creative part of your awareness.

Mental uses This essential oil helps you maintain focus and aids you in staying grounded. Use it to dissipate scattered energy and negative thoughtforms, as well as to deflect negative energy. This oil clears out the deeper recesses of your mind, and when used with intention, ravensara aids in breaking up resistant repetitive thoughts. Ultimately, it helps quiet your mind and call forth inner peace.

Emotional uses Ravensara can be used to help you during emotional crisis. Just as it aids in strengthening your physical immune system, it works similarly to strengthen your emotional immune system, enhancing your ability to fight off energetic emotional strain and patterns buried deep within. Use this when negative emotions wreak havoc in your life. It scrambles and releases your unconscious broadcast of programs that perpetuate negative patterns.

Physical uses Ravensara is the oil of choice for warding off germs that affect the respiratory system. Use this oil to relieve sinus and bronchial congestion and clear bacterial infections. This antiviral oil is powerful to dissipate the potential for stubborn viral attacks due to its strong immunological qualities. Use it with eucalyptus, tea tree, and clove for a powerful synergistic blend to fight colds and flu. Ravensara is a good aromatherapy ally for caregivers, dental professionals, ear/nose/throat specialists, healthcare practitioners, housekeepers, infectious disease specialists, manicurists, nurses, podiatrists, pulmonary specialists, and shamanic practitioners.

Therapeutic properties Analgesic, antibacterial, antibiotic, antiseptic, antispasmodic, antitoxic, antitussive, antiviral, carminative, cholagogic, choleretic, diuretic, febrifugal, sedative, stimulative, tonic.

Divine guidance Is your mind carrying around toxic memories? Are you ingesting unhealthy foods that contain immune-weakening toxins? It's time to take the necessary steps to rid your mind of toxic thoughts. It is time to release old memories that are interfering with your ability to be happy. Use your powers of intuition to find guidance that you require.

For your safety Do not use if pregnant or nursing.

> **Interesting tidbits:**
> In Madagascar, ravensara seeds are called clove nutmeg, although it is not the same as traditional nutmeg. In *Essential Aromatherapy*, Worwood states that ravensara bark is used to make a certain type of rum.

ROSE
All That Is

BOTANICAL NAME	*Rosa damascena*
NOTE	base to middle
METHOD OF EXTRACTION	steam distillation
PARTS USED	flowers
FRAGRANCE	deep, floral, sweet
COLOR(S)	pink, red, white
CHAKRA(S)	heart
ASTROLOGICAL SIGN(S)	Cancer, Virgo, Libra, Taurus
PLANET(S)	Pluto, Venus
NUMBER(S)	0, 4
ANIMAL(S)	dove, swan, unicorn
ELEMENT(S)	all

Affirmation I am love. All that surrounds me and all that is attracted to me is love. I look within and love all aspects of myself exactly as I am. I attract love, joy, and happiness into my life, and I am comforted. Blessings are always present. I have an entourage of angels and spirit guides at my beck and call.

Complementary flower essences Holly to heal from a breakup and to encourage self-love and compassion. *Honeysuckle* to encourage happiness and love. *Olive* to inspire rest and rejuvenation. *Water Violet* to maintain a stronger connection with others.

Complementary stones Danburite, kunzite, pink calcite, rhodonite, rhodochrosite, rose quartz.

About the plant Damask rose grows as a bush that reaches various heights up to 7 feet with fragrant pink or light red flowers with many petals.

Chemical components Phenylethanol, citronellol, alkanes and alkenes, geraniol, nerol, eugenol, farnesol, terpinen, methyl eugenol.

Spiritual uses Rose is a reminder that love is the answer to all. Use rose to radiate love in a wide circumference around your being. With the heart chakra being the center of your consciousness, love is who you truly are. Rose is helpful in your meditation practice for expanding your sphere of love. Use rose oil to petition aid from Saint Therese of Lisieux to help manifest miracles. Rose oil is associated with your guardian angels, Mother Mary, Our Lady of Guadalupe, Kuan Yin (the goddess of mercy and compassion), and the Archangels Chamuel, Gabriel, Haniel, and Metatron. This essential oil assists in bringing back good memories and the pure teachings of Atlantis.

Mental uses Rose helps you maintain your focus and attention on your heart chakra and love. Imagine all that you are, all that you do, and all you attract is love as you allow this aroma to permeate your energy field.

Emotional uses Roses symbolize love and beauty. Rose helps you attract healthy, romantic relationships as well as supportive, loving friendships and good business colleagues. Keeping this aroma in your field encourages kindness, compassion, and tolerance. It also reduces stress and worry and helps relieve anxiety and the symptoms of depression. Use rose when you need to nurture yourself. Rose encourages joy and happiness.

Physical uses Rose is known for its use in skin care for regeneration and reduction of scars, wrinkles, and stretch marks. Because of its nurturing and calming influence on the mind and emotions, rose is beneficial to reduce inflammation and blood pressure. Rose is a good aromatherapy ally for angel communicators, beekeepers, cardiologists, clairvoyants, dermatologists, estheticians, marriage counselors, mothers, sex therapists, and wedding planners.

Therapeutic properties Astringent, cholagogic, digestive, diuretic, hepatic, rejuvenative (skin scars and stretch marks), tonic, vasodilator.

Divine guidance Are you looking for more love in your life? You are good at giving love and can open even more to receive loving, supportive friends and family in your life. You are ready to increase the love in your life as well as the miracles that occur all around you. Determine how you want to be loved and start out by loving yourself in that way.

For your safety No known contraindications. It is best not to use during the first trimester of pregnancy.

> ### Interesting tidbits:
> This plant is also known as cabbage rose or French rose. The tenth-century Arab physician Avicenna was purportedly the first to distill rose oil. It takes 65 pounds of petals to make one ounce of rose oil! Interestingly, the petals must be harvested before sunrise. Roses traditionally symbolize a happy marriage, which is why they are often used in wedding bouquets. The scent of rose is associated with Mother Mary, as the scent or manifestations of roses are commonly reported in association with her Divine appearances.

ROSEMARY
Mental Acuity

BOTANICAL NAME	*Rosmarinus officinalis*
NOTE	middle
METHOD OF EXTRACTION	steam distillation
PARTS USED	flowers and leaves
FRAGRANCE	clean, crisp, herbal, penetrating, resinous, strong
COLOR(S)	blue-green
CHAKRA(S)	crown, third eye
ASTROLOGICAL SIGN(S)	Virgo
PLANET(S)	Mars, Mercury, Uranus
NUMBER(S)	1, 11
ANIMAL(S)	dog, elephant, fox, hawk, owl
ELEMENT(S)	air, fire

Affirmation I am clear, energized, and connected. I am grateful for all my creative and business skills. I earn unlimited income doing what I love. I have great mental clarity. It is easy for me to awaken my consciousness and be fully present in my daily activities. I am grounded and focused.

Complementary flower essences Chestnut Bud to recognize and benefit from patterns or past mistakes. *Crab Apple* for self-acceptance. *Mustard* to fill yourself with lightness as you remove negative vibes.

Complementary stones Citrine, clear quartz, tabular quartz, emerald, malachite, Orthoceras fossil, rainbow obsidian, scolecite, time link quartz crystal.

About the plant Rosemary is a hardy evergreen shrub with linear leaves and tiny pale-blue flowers that reaches a height of about 2 to 6 feet.

Chemical components Cineole, borneol, camphor, verbenone, pinene, bornyl acetate, linalool, camphene, caryophyllene, terpineol, cymene, curcumene, nonanol, terpinen.

Spiritual uses Rosemary helps you with your spiritual memory and focus. Use rosemary to awaken your spiritual consciousness. The ancient energy of rosemary provides a deeper understanding through memory retrieval of previous incarnations. Use it during regression therapy to capitalize on memories of the past and the lessons learned. Add rosemary to a synergistic blend to clear out negative energy in general and before your spiritual practices. Use rosemary to connect with Archangel Sabrael to release jealousy.

Mental uses Rosemary brings mental clarity and sharpness. Use it during times of study for retention of information. Smell rosemary oil to help you recall information during tests. This fragrant oil especially helps with mental acuity regarding business transactions. Rosemary is helpful for the elderly to encourage mental alertness, memory, and to be more present in daily activities.

Emotional uses Rosemary is beneficial for deflecting negativity and jealousy. Use it to help clear out negative emotions and paranoia. Rosemary helps you to attract loyal and authentic friends and romantic relationships and weed out those who are untrustworthy. Rosemary is useful for healing emotions by encouraging them to come to the surface. Rosemary will help release outdated beliefs, balance karma, and delete molecular memory to help you become healthy, whole, and complete. This oil can help during the grieving process by encouraging positive memories to ensue with the realization that the memory of your loved ones never dies.

Physical uses Rosemary kills germs and is a good disinfectant that protects against contagious diseases. Use this oil to open your airways and improve the depth of your breathing. Rosemary is well known for its skin and health-care benefits. It stimulates the scalp and can be used as an aid to prevent baldness. Add to a synergistic blend intended to repel insects. Rosemary is a good aromatherapy ally for accountants, chefs, ear/nose/throat specialists, environmentalists, hairstylists, law enforcement professionals, librarians, marriage counselors, neurologists, pest control professionals, and wedding planners.

Therapeutic properties Analgesic, antibacterial, antidepressant, antifungal, antineuralgic, antioxidant, antiparasitic, antirheumatic, antiseptic, antispasmodic, antitoxic, antitussive, antiviral, aphrodisiac, astringent, carminative, cephalic, cholagogic, choleretic, cicatrizant, cytophylactic, decongestant, detoxifier, diaphoretic, digestive, diuretic, emmenagogic, hepatic, hypertensor, insecticidal (strong), invigorating, laxative, nervine, rejuvenative (skin cells), rubefacient, stimulative (adrenal glands and nerves), stomachic, sudorific, tonic, vulnerary, warming.

Divine guidance Do you need more mental clarity? Are you asking the question, "Why is this happening to me?" Are you caught in a pattern in which you are experiencing the same situation over and over again? Now is a good time to look into regression to uncover the original sources of the issues presently at play in your life. Activate your inner entrepreneur through focused study. Use your acquired knowledge to reach your goals.

For your safety Avoid use in cases of hypertension. Avoid if prone to epileptic seizures.

Interesting tidbits:

In Spain and Italy, rosemary was used as protection from witchcraft. This herb is associated with the muse Mnemosyne, whose name means "memory," and Minerva, the Roman goddess of wisdom and knowledge. Rosemary has become a symbol of loyalty and fidelity. Historically, it has been used to lace wedding bouquets. This Mediterranean herb has been used to complement culinary dishes for thousands of years.

ROSEWOOD
Spiritual Magnificence

BOTANICAL NAME	*Aniba rosaeodora*
NOTE	top to middle to base
METHOD OF EXTRACTION	steam distillation
PARTS USED	wood
FRAGRANCE	floral, mild, rosy, soft, sweet, woody
COLOR(S)	brown, olive green, yellow
CHAKRA(S)	heart, solar plexus
ASTROLOGICAL SIGN(S)	Leo, Sagittarius
PLANET(S)	Jupiter, Sun
NUMBER(S)	7
ANIMAL(S)	dragonfly, hawk, lion
ELEMENT(S)	water

Affirmation I focus on all my good attributes and amplify them. I have the courage to step forward with joy and enthusiasm. I radiate my magnificence. I am self-confident. My value and worth are recognized by others and by myself. I am a money magnet.

Complementary flower essences Elm to aid with the focus on the present moment and self-worth. *Mustard* to relieve depression. *White Chestnut* to release the repetitive thoughts that prevent inner peace and self-confidence.

Complementary stones Citrine, golden topaz, heliodor, kunzite, lepidolite, purple-dyed agate, sunstone.

About the plant Rosewood is an evergreen tree that reaches heights of more than 100 feet; it is found in the tropics of America, the West Indies, and the tropical rainforests of Brazil.

Chemical components Linalool, terpineol, linalool oxide, cineol.

Spiritual uses Rosewood supports you in your intention to increase your connection with the Divine and to maximize your intuitive skills, including the sensory gifts of clairvoyance, clairaudience, claircognizance, and clairsentience. Inhale rosewood as a reminder of the miracle worker within you and your inborn spiritual magnificence. It helps you connect with a strong sense of self so you can actualize your Divine spark.

Mental uses In combination with bergamot and lemon, rosewood makes an excellent trinity of oils to improve mental clarity and a joyful outlook on life. It helps raise you out of depression (as an adjunct to other therapies) and renew your self-confidence. Use it to improve your courage to put good thoughts into action. As you become consciously aware of your thoughts with the help of this oil, you can discard outdated thoughts and replace them with thoughts that focus on the life you want to live.

Emotional uses Rosewood increases joyfulness and self-esteem and is helpful for relieving the symptoms of depression. It relieves stress and aids in rehabilitation after periods of weakness to stimulate and rejuvenate. Rosewood increases your courage to embrace the magnificent person you truly are. It is also advantageous when you are trying to absorb all that is going on in your life and the lives of those around you. Rosewood oil encourages feelings of worthiness in loving and romantic relationships.

Physical uses Rosewood helps to relieve the symptoms of depression and mental illness stemming from mood swings. Rosewood, an antifungal essential oil, is beneficial to fight candida. Rosewood oil amplifies the vital life force within you. It promotes passionate action toward a goal with the motivation required to get things done. Operating in the physical world requires money and vitality, so with this oil as your ally, align yourself with the vibration of the resources you require to move forward with a project or plan. Rosewood is a good aromatherapy ally for bankers, brokers, builders, counselors, inventors, life coaches, marriage counselors, pest control professionals, psychologists, and wedding planners.

Therapeutic properties Analgesic, antibacterial, anticonvulsive, antidepressant, antifungal, antiparasitic, antiseptic (throat), antiviral, aphrodisiac, calmative, cephalic, deodorizer, emollient (skin), euphoriant, insecticidal, regenerative (skin tissue), stimulative (immune system), tonic, uplifting.

Divine guidance Have you been feeling down in the dumps? Do you need to add a bit of jazziness to your life? Do you need some brilliance and enthusiasm? This is a time of prosperity and purpose. You are ready to step into your power and be all that you were meant to be. You are aligned with the magnificence and the courage to show yourself in your fullest splendor!

For your safety No known contraindications.

> **Interesting tidbits:**
> Prior to the widespread distillation, rosewood wood chips were used as fuel for fire at distilleries. Rosewood has been used to make canoes by indigenous people of Brazil. The scent of the wood chips is reminiscent of the spring flower lily of the valley.

SAGE
Scrubbing Bubbles

BOTANICAL NAME	*Salvia officinalis*
NOTE	top
METHOD OF EXTRACTION	steam distillation
PARTS USED	leaves, flowers, and buds
FRAGRANCE	camphoraceous, fresh, green, pungent, strong, sweet, woody
COLOR(S)	brown, green, lavender, yellow
CHAKRA(S)	root, navel, solar plexus
ASTROLOGICAL SIGN(S)	Scorpio
PLANET(S)	Moon, Pluto
NUMBER(S)	16/7
ANIMAL(S)	snake, turtle
ELEMENT(S)	earth, fire

Affirmation I am safe and sound. I am out of harm's way. All is well. I surround myself with trustworthy people. I am blessed, and I am always divinely protected. I am enveloped in a sphere of goodness and well-being.

Complementary flower essences Mimulus for oversensitivity to energy. *Rescue Remedy* for fears. *Red Chestnut* when you can't overcome the fear that something bad will happen.

Complementary stones Amethyst, ametrine, brown agate, golden calcite, green moss agate, green tourmaline, hematite, jet, lapis lazuli, rainbow obsidian, smoky quartz, snowflake obsidian, tourmalinated quartz, vanadinite.

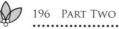

About the plant Sage is a Mediterranean evergreen plant that grows up to 3 feet with grayish green leaves and small lavender-colored flowers.

Chemical components Camphor, thujone, borneol, cineole, caryophyllene, camphene, pinene, bornyl acetate, pinene.

Spiritual uses Sage is the ultimate go-to oil for clearing out negative energy from your space and your personal energy field. Use sage to ground your spiritual practice into your everyday life. Keep it close by for protection while doing readings or any type of spiritual healing. This oil provides the ever-important mindfulness, awareness, and peripheral vision in spiritual practice.

Mental uses Sage oil helps you transform the mental composition of your thoughts, so use sage to help you restructure thoughts and give them new life with a positive twist. On a vibrational level, use it to break down old, repetitive ways of thinking and let yourself reconstitute them with a new flair. Sage helps you to resonate with wisdom and inspiration and to recognize the difference between wisdom and knowledge.

Emotional uses Use sage with the intention of shaking out emotional states that have been firmly established in the navel and root chakras. Instead of total disintegration, sage destabilizes the negativity associated with challenging memories or experiences. Therefore, this oil helps you reintegrate the lessons captured from the experience, making you a much more powerful person because of it. Sage reduces anxiety and raises your vibration. It helps to relieve symptoms of depression.

Physical uses Sage has been used throughout the ages to balance female reproductive hormones to eliminate or reduce the challenges of infertility, premenstrual syndrome, and menopause. Sage is a stimulant, increases cerebral blood flow, and potentially raises low blood pressure. Sage oil can be used to reduce excessive perspiration. It also minimizes lactation in nursing mothers. Sage is a good aromatherapy ally for chefs, clairvoyants, counselors, doulas, ghost hunters, gynecologists, intuitive readers, judges, law enforcement officers, librarians, meditation practitioners/facilitators, musicians, neurologists, New Age retailers, phlebotomists, psychologists, Reiki practitioners, shamanic practitioners, spiritual counselors, and spiritual healers.

Therapeutic properties Antibacterial, antidepressant, antidiabetic, antifungal, antigalactagogic, anti-inflammatory, antioxidant, antiparasitic, antirheumatic, antiseptic, antispasmodic, antisudorific, antitussive, antiviral, aperitive, astringent, blood purifier, carminative, cholagogic, cicatrizant, depurative, digestive, disinfectant (strong), diuretic, emmenagogic, estrogenic, euphoriant, febrifugal, hemostatic (bleeding gums), hepatic, hypertensor, insecticidal, laxative, nervine, stimulative (brain, circulatory system, adrenal glands), stomachic, tonic (digestive system), vulnerary, warming.

Divine guidance Do you fear betrayal or feel threatened in some way? Are you perhaps surrounded by negative or untrustworthy people or find yourself in questionable situations? Focus your intention on deflecting the negativity, surround yourself in a loving cloak of protection, and know that your angels and other spirit guides are watching out for you.

For your safety Could have adverse effects on the central nervous system. Do not use if pregnant or nursing.

Interesting tidbits:

Just as its name implies, sage carries the vibration of wisdom. Throughout history, sage was consumed not only for its pleasant taste but also in the belief that it would bring wisdom to those who ate it. Sage leaves were used for wart removal in the seventeenth century. Sage has been burned in purification ceremonies for thousands of years. This herb has been known to ward off evil since ancient times. This is also considered an essential cooking herb, along with parsley, rosemary, and thyme, as made popular in the song "Scarborough Fair."

SANDALWOOD
Prayer, Contemplation, and Wisdom

BOTANICAL NAME	*Santalum album*
NOTE	base
METHOD OF EXTRACTION	steam distillation
PARTS USED	inner wood
FRAGRANCE	exotic, lingering, subtle, woody
COLOR(S)	the full spectrum
CHAKRA(S)	all
ASTROLOGICAL SIGN(S)	Aquarius, Pisces
PLANET(S)	Neptune, Uranus
NUMBER(S)	9, 822
ANIMAL(S)	elephant, hawk, mouse, white buffalo
ELEMENT(S)	air, water

Affirmation My head and my heart are aligned with the Divine. I am a miracle worker. I spread love and well-being to all beings. I am balanced, aligned, healthy, and strong. It is easy for me to stand in the center of my power and emanate love. I open myself up to the healing energy of the love and prayers that people are sending to me and focus on sending out prayers and well-being to all beings in need.

Complementary flower essences Gorse to improve your faith and optimism. *Holly* to release hurt feelings and jealousy while improving kindness in words and deeds. *Impatiens* for tolerance and patience with self and others.

Complementary stones Amethyst, amethyst druzy, angelite, clear quartz, howlite, jade, pink tourmaline, rhodochrosite, selenite, serpentine.

About the plant Sandalwood is an Asian evergreen tree that reaches heights of about 30 feet; it has small flowers that produce fruits.

Chemical components Santalol, bisabolol, nuciferol, farnesol, dendrolasin, bergamotol, bulnesol, lanceolol, nerolidol, guaiol, curcumene, santalene.

Spiritual uses Sandalwood is well-loved for its benefits during meditation, as it elicits a quiet mind. Its fragrance has been used in Buddhist and Hindu religious ceremonies and is used regularly in metaphysical, spiritual, and yogic practices. Mala beads, or prayer beads, are often made of sandalwood. Sandalwood helps you align with the vibrational essence of Buddha and Kuan Yin (goddess of mercy and compassion). Sandalwood helps you to improve your faith and confidence in spiritual pursuits. It aids in believing in the power of prayer.

Mental uses Sandalwood induces a calm and quiet mind. It helps align mental processes toward self-improvement, self-actualization, and self-acceptance. Sandalwood is a tool to activate the wise scholar within and the intellect from a place of wisdom. It is beneficial for clearing your thoughts of anything that is not resonating at the vibration of love.

Emotional uses Sandalwood helps to align you with compassion, inner peace, tolerance, and love. It tells you to love yourself and others completely and wholly just as you are! This oil helps you get in touch with positive ways to integrate situations and emotions into your life. Use it to help you get to the source of what's eating at you and achieve a new, lighter perspective.

Physical uses Sandalwood is a good fixative in synergistic blends as it helps to stabilize the aroma. Use sandalwood for infections of the chest, throat, and bladder. Use it to relieve nervous tension, stress, and anxiety for overall energetic healing of all types of illness. Sandalwood helps to rebalance the body to recover from nervous exhaustion. Sandalwood is an aromatherapy ally for meditation facilitators/practitioners, mystics, sex therapists, visionary leaders, and therapists, especially practitioners of emotional freedom technique (EFT), or tapping, a therapeutic psychological tool to heal emotional stress.

Therapeutic properties Analgesic, antibacterial, antidepressant, antifungal, anti-infectious, anti-inflammatory, antiphlogistic, antipruritic, antiseptic, antispasmodic, antistress, antitussive, antiviral, aphrodisiac, astringent, calmative, carminative, cicatrizant, decongestant, deodorizer, diaphoretic, diuretic, emollient, euphoriant, febrifugal, fixative, insecticidal, relaxant, sedative, stimulative, stomachic, tonic.

Divine guidance Are you reaching out in prayer asking for help? Are you in touch with your connection with all life—the seen and unseen? Tap into your innate ability to intuit whatever you need whenever you need it. Acknowledge your intuition and trust your awareness of your own feelings as well as the feelings of others.

For your safety No known contraindications.

> **Interesting tidbits:**
> One of the oldest aromatic woods known, sandalwood is mentioned in Vedic literature dating back to 500–300 BC. It is the archetypal scent of India, whose Sanskrit name is *chandana*. This wood is resistant to termites. Ancient Egyptians used sandalwood in the embalming process.

SPIKENARD
The Feminine Christ

BOTANICAL NAME	*Nardostachys jatamansi*
NOTE	middle to base
METHOD OF EXTRACTION	steam distillation
PARTS USED	roots
FRAGRANCE	earthy, heavy, musty, peaty, valerian root–like; reminiscent of dirty socks
COLOR(S)	pastel blue, navy blue, brown, green, magenta, turquoise
CHAKRA(S)	root, crown
ASTROLOGICAL SIGN(S)	Aquarius, Pisces, Virgo
PLANET(S)	Juno, Neptune, Uranus, Venus
NUMBER(S)	7
ANIMAL(S)	dragonfly, fish
ELEMENT(S)	earth

Affirmation I am love. I align my consciousness with gentleness, compassion, and goodwill toward all. My focus is on kindness. I make it my goal and intention to have compassion and tolerance and to live love. I am aligned with the healing powers of inner peace and empathy. I am able to help others by vibrating love through my presence, words, and actions.

Complementary flower essences Chestnut Bud to release worrisome thoughts and improve sleep. *Vervain* for high tension and hyperactivity. *Vine* to calm aggressiveness and improve compassion and kindness.

Complementary stones Angelite, blue calcite, blue chalcedony, celestite, chrysocolla, dumortierite, magenta-dyed agate.

About the plant Native to Asia and the Himalayas, found at an altitude of 9,000–15,000 feet, spikenard is a flowering plant with pink bell-shaped flowers that reaches a height of about 2 feet.

Chemical components Nardol, formic acid, selinene, dihydro ionone, nardol isomer, selinene isomer, propionic acid, caryophyllene, cubebol, gurjunene, hexadecene, nerolidol, calamenene, epoxy-ledene.

Spiritual uses Use spikenard to remind you to be receptive to your intuition and to accept the part of yourself that is able to imagine a better way of life for all beings. Spikenard can help highly intuitive people deal with incoming energies. Through spikenard's calming vibes, inner peace and personal self-care are possible even when dealing with the challenging vibrations of others. Archetypes for this oil are Christ, Mother Mary, Kuan Yin, Isis, and Mary Magdalene. The associated Archangels are Tzaphkiel and Uriel. Use this oil to awaken your awareness of your spiritual purpose. This essential oil assists in aligning with the pure teachings of Atlantis.

Mental uses The archetypal energy of spikenard embodies compassion, inner peace, nurturing, and great wisdom. Through meditation with this oil as an ally, you can begin to grasp the difference between information, knowledge, and wisdom. This oil is a reminder that when you strive for wisdom, information and knowledge will always be available. The calming vibration of this essential oil slows inner self-talk to help you sort out the many mental images and conversations going on inside.

Emotional uses Spikenard helps to calm and balance your emotions, thereby increasing your emotional maturity. Spikenard brings composure to turbulent emotions like hysteria, anger, hostility, and irritability. It promotes feelings of kindness and compassion. This oil is a reminder of the Divine Mother within, who hears and knows truth and accepts you unconditionally.

Use spikenard to amplify retribution, both positive and negative. Utilize this oil's energy to amplify your intention through your heart and the thymus (the upper heart).

Physical uses Spikenard is a sedative. It relaxes the muscles, helps you sleep, and reduces anxiety and physical tension. Also known as nard, this oil aids in overcoming birth difficulties. The healing effect of this oil relieves stress-related conditions, which have been said to be the source of all illness and disease. Spikenard encourages hair growth. This oil acts as a fixative to stabilize the volatile oils in blends. Spikenard is a good aromatherapy ally for acupuncturists, angel communicators, aromatherapists, body workers, chiropractors, clairvoyants, hairstylists, heart surgeons, hospice caregivers, insomnia specialists, intuitive readers, lawyers, librarians, mothers, mystics, neurologists, parents, and visionary leaders.

Therapeutic properties Analgesic, antibacterial, antibiotic, anticonvulsive, antifungal, anti-inflammatory, antioxidant, antiparasitic, antiseptic, antispasmodic, aperitive, calmative, cardiotonic, carminative, deodorizer, depurative, digestive, diuretic, emmenagogic, febrifugal, hepatic, laxative, nervine, sedative, tonic.

Divine guidance Are you trying to comprehend all that is going on around you? Are you in the process of recovering from a time of upset or emotional challenge? Seek out calming experiences such as mediation. Take notice of the signs and symbols around you and contemplate their meaning.

For your safety Do not use if pregnant or nursing.

> **Interesting tidbits:**
> Spikenard has been used as a sleep aid and muscle relaxant for thousands of years. It is part of the valerian family and is also known as muskroot. Some historical accounts state that spikenard was the oil in the alabaster jar used by Mary Magdalene on the feet of Jesus the Christ, to prepare him for torture.

SPRUCE
Peaceful Life

BOTANICAL NAME	*Tsuga canadensis*
NOTE	middle
METHOD OF EXTRACTION	steam distillation
PARTS USED	bark and branches
FRAGRANCE	balsamic, green, invigorating, pine-like, sweet, woody
COLOR(S)	blue, blue-green, green, white
CHAKRA(S)	heart, third eye, crown
ASTROLOGICAL SIGN(S)	Gemini, Sagittarius
PLANET(S)	Mars, Mercury
NUMBER(S)	888
ANIMAL(S)	elephant, elk, white buffalo
ELEMENT(S)	air

Affirmation I am calm. I am at peace. I am relaxed. All is well. I live a spiritual, peaceful life. I am a conduit for goodness, prosperity, and love. I easily transform anger and frustration to align with tranquility and inner peace through conscious release and awareness. I enjoy relaxing in nature to regenerate and rejuvenate my energy field.

Complementary flower essences Oak to rejuvenate from exhaustion. *Red Chestnut* to clear worrisome thoughts. *Wild Oat* to gain clarity on your life purpose.

Complementary stones Azurite-malachite, chrysocolla, chrysoprase, lapis lazuli, seraphinite, sodalite.

About the plant Spruce is a blue-green-needled evergreen tree that reaches heights of up to 200 feet.

Chemical components Pinene, bornyl acetate, limonene, camphene, myrcene, carene, camphor, borneol.

Spiritual uses Spruce helps you to channel the higher wisdom and knowledge of the universe while maintaining a grounded connection with the physical world. It aligns your consciousness with Christ Consciousness and the return of light to the planet. Use it at your third eye and crown chakras during meditation. Allow this oil to be your ally when doing shamanic journeywork or engaging in deep meditative practices. The symbolic and vibrational energy of this oil links your heart and mind with the spiritual realm. Use it to call upon Archangel Camael to realign angry and aggressive feelings with their opposite, positive counterparts.

Mental uses Spruce helps you to gain greater perspective by becoming aware of how the words you speak affect your health, allowing you to employ "word patrol" to uncover sources of imbalance and disease. Use self-observation to transform your thinking. Spruce encourages clear thinking, creativity, and great ideas. Just like the colors blue and green reduce inflamed thinking, this essential oil calms and relieves stress.

Emotional uses Spruce oil helps you recognize the evolution of your emotions and spirit as they travel through time and experience. Find your way to euphoria and bliss with the green, clean scent of spruce oil. Spruce inspires getting in touch with feelings through clarity and vibrations of strength and safety. It aligns you with comfort and joy energetically. Use spruce as a heart and mind connector, which contributes to balanced emotions.

Physical uses Spruce provides a feeling of stamina and endurance. Inhale spruce deeply to open up the respiratory system and to clear the sinuses and all the breathing pathways. The anti-inflammatory vibrations of this oil balance your physical body to restore health and well-being through release of stress. Spruce is a good aromatherapy ally for ear/nose/throat specialists, housekeepers, mental health counselors, mystics, librarians, life coaches, pulmonary specialists, shamanic practitioners, and visionary leaders.

Therapeutic properties Anti-inflammatory, antiparasitic, antiseptic, antispasmodic, antitussive, astringent, diaphoretic, diuretic, hemostatic, nervine, rubefacient, sedative, tonic, vulnerary, warming.

Divine guidance Are you dealing with an inflamed or unbalanced situation—physically, mentally, spiritually, or emotionally? Have you been challenged by imbalances in your body? Take steps to balance your emotions through journaling, exercise, and healthy communication. Nurture yourself through rest and by taking good care of your body, mind, and spirit. Yoga and meditation are beneficial. Take notice of the signs and symbols around you and contemplate their meaning.

For your safety Spruce is a possible skin irritant depending on the plant species.

Interesting tidbits:
Spruce tree cones were used as incense in the winter and to encourage happiness. Spruce resin was burned with other herbs during Nordic Christmas festivities. Branches of spruce, along with other evergreens, make a perfect centerpiece on the dining table during the winter holidays.

 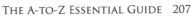

Sweet Marjoram
Breathe Deeply and Know All Is Well

Botanical name	*Origanum majorana*
Note	middle
Method of extraction	steam distillation
Parts used	flowering tops and leaves
Fragrance	herbaceous, medicinal, penetrating, slightly spicy, warm
Color(s)	black, dark blue, magenta, purple
Chakra(s)	crown, heart, navel, throat, third eye
Astrological sign(s)	Taurus, Libra, Scorpio
Planet(s)	Ceres, Jupiter, Mercury
Number(s)	8, 822
Animal(s)	dog, dove, horse
Element(s)	earth, air

Affirmation I am safe. I have constant protection surrounding me, deflecting anything not for my highest good. I have the courage and self-confidence to create my world. My emotions are balanced. I am clear and joyful. Events from my past positively affect my present and future; I have released any negative emotional charge the past may have contained.

Complementary flower essences Cherry Plum for when the burdens of life are so intense that you feel like you'll have a nervous breakdown. *Rescue Remedy* for immediate relief of hysteria or trauma. *Star of Bethlehem* for shock and stress.

Complementary stones Black tourmaline, cobaltoan calcite, emerald, jet, kyanite, magenta-dyed agate, pink calcite, red tiger's eye, smoky quartz.

About the plant Sweet marjoram is a bushy Mediterranean plant with light green leaves and white or purple flowers that reaches a height of about 2 feet.

Chemical components Terpinen, sabinene hydrate, linalyl acetate, terpinene, terpineol, sabinene, cymene, linalool, terpinolene.

Spiritual uses Sweet marjoram helps you to release subconscious fears and reminds you of your faith. Use it to call upon Archangel Auriel to help release worries, negative thoughts, and fears; Archangel Jophiel for inner wisdom and beauty; and Archangel Michael for protection. By calling on the goddess of love and beauty, Aphrodite, sweet marjoram helps you align your spiritual heart and mind to align your crown and heart chakras to attract your spiritual romantic partner (but keep in mind that it is an anaphrodisiac). This essential oil also assists in bringing back good memories and the pure teachings of Atlantis.

Mental uses Sweet marjoram relaxes the mental body enough to release the grasp on repetitive and/or negative thoughts associated with fears, phobias, and obsessions. Sweet marjoram also helps you speak your truth with love and beauty.

Emotional uses Sweet marjoram calms hysteria and quiets the emotions enough to sort out what you are feeling. It helps release paranoia and fears—both known and unknown—and helps strengthen your belief in yourself. Use sweet marjoram to shore up inner strength and courage when you are feeling emotionally weak and vulnerable. In *The Fragrant Mind*, Worwood states that marjoram aids in healing addiction to alcohol, soothes aggression, relieves delirium, quiet fits of hysteria, and helps release phobias.

Physical uses Sweet marjoram is bedtime's favorite friend to encourage healthy breathing and deep, healing sleep. Inhale the vapors to relax and release the day. Sweet marjoram relieves headaches and sinus congestion, and opens breathing passageways to relieve symptoms of bronchitis and pneumonia. Sweet marjoram lowers blood pressure. Use it to calm the sting of insect bites. Sweet marjoram is a good aromatherapy ally for athletes, counselors, drug rehabilitation specialists, ear/nose/throat specialists, Feng Shui practitioners, ghost hunters, insomnia specialists, law enforcement professionals, lawyers, marathon participants, marriage counselors, pulmonary specialists, travel professionals, and wedding planners.

Therapeutic properties Analgesic, anaphrodisiac, antibacterial, antifungal, antioxidant, antiseptic, antispasmodic, antistress, antitussive, antiviral, calmative, carminative, cephalic, cordial, decongestant, detoxifier, diaphoretic, digestive, diuretic, emmenagogic, febrifugal, galactagogic, hypotensor, laxative, nervine, restorative, sedative, stomachic, tonic (heart), vasodilator (arterial), vulnerary, warming.

Divine guidance Are you in love? Are you focused on romance right now? Decide to create happiness and harmony. You'll start to see an increase in loyal and caring friends in your life—as soon as you decide you are willing to accept the love in your life. Allow the development of a new romantic relationship or the rekindling of an existing one.

For your safety Avoid in cases of low blood pressure. Do not use if pregnant or nursing.

> ### Interesting tidbits:
> According to Greek mythology, Aphrodite is credited with bringing sweet marjoram into creation. Its use in Egypt dates back to 1000 BC. Both the Greeks and Romans crowned couples with sweet marjoram at their weddings. Dried marjoram was used in pillows in Medieval Europe to encourage sleep.

TEA TREE
Clean and Clear

BOTANICAL NAME	*Melaleuca alternifolia*
NOTE	top to middle
METHOD OF EXTRACTION	steam distillation
PARTS USED	leaves
FRAGRANCE	clean, disinfectant-like, herbaceous, medicinal, spicy, strong
COLOR(S)	green, white, yellow
CHAKRA(S)	heart, third eye, throat
ASTROLOGICAL SIGN(S)	Aquarius
PLANET(S)	Uranus
NUMBER(S)	11, 222
ANIMAL(S)	dolphin, hawk
ELEMENT(S)	air

Affirmation I consciously request and accept the help of my angels and other spirit guides. My life flows easily with grace. The energy of healing, love, and well-being flows through me. Meditation is a normal part of my day. My crown, third eye, and throat chakras are balanced and aligned. My intuition is intact.

Complementary flower essences Crab Apple to relieve feelings of being contaminated or infected. *Gorse* to revitalize faith and to heal from illness. *Star of Bethlehem* for recovery after a shock.

 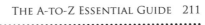

Complementary stones Angelite, aragonite, blue lace agate, blue tiger's eye, blue chalcedony, blue or green onyx, dogtooth calcite, orange calcite, sodalite, turquoise.

About the plant Tea tree is an evergreen tree that reaches a height of up to 25 feet. It has papery bark and white flowers.

Chemical components Terpinen, terpinene, terpinolene, cineole, terpineol, cymene, pinene, sabinene, aromadendrene, ledene, cadinene, viridiflorol, limonene, globulol.

Spiritual uses Tea tree facilitates the download and processing of Divine inspiration, healing light, and true wisdom. It is especially beneficial for guiding your higher consciousness to be a Divine channel of God's love and to connect with Archangel Gabriel to open your spiritual gift of clairaudience. Tea tree's crisp aroma brings mindfulness to your daily life, which aids in the spiritual practice of self-observation. Use tea tree with the intention to grasp the significance of karma, cause and effect, retribution, and the spiritual consequences and benefits of action or lack of action.

Mental uses Use tea tree with conscious intent to conduct incoming and outgoing wisdom, vibrations, and communication, including mind-to-mind communication. Tea tree can help restore your senses after a shock.

Emotional uses Tea tree encourages expansiveness in experiencing the depth of your emotions. It opens your heart and diaphragm in order to embrace and accept your feelings, and then to clear out any toxic feelings, allowing you to be free and present in all your relationships.

Physical uses Tea tree is useful for healing infections. It has strong antiseptic qualities and is recognized for its anti-infectious and antifungal qualities. Use before and after an operation to improve the immune system as it is effective as an antiviral and germicidal agent. It is especially beneficial for the relief of a sore throat, toothache, earache, and sinus conditions. Tea tree has calmed the sting of an insect bite and has been known to expel intestinal parasites. Tea tree is a good aromatherapy ally for dental professionals, dermatologists, ear/nose/throat specialists, housekeepers, infectious disease specialists, lawyers, manicurists, mothers, nurses, podiatrists, pulmonary specialists, and speakers.

Therapeutic properties Analgesic, antibacterial, antibiotic, antimicrobial, anti-inflammatory, antiparasitic, antipruritic, antiseptic (strong), antitussive, antiviral, carminative, cicatrizant, cordial, decongestant, diaphoretic, insecticidal, refreshing, revitalizing, stimulative, sudorific, vulnerary.

Divine guidance Are you looking at something from only one angle? Do you need to rise above a situation to find truth and see with greater clarity? It is time to take steps to gain a new perspective on life. The time has come to believe in your choices and know that they are good. Trust your ability to see things and read situations clearly.

For your safety Possible skin irritant.

Interesting tidbits:
Because of its papery bark, tea tree is part of a grouping of trees known as paperbarks. The qualities and value of tea tree have been well-recognized by the Aborigines of Australia for many centuries.

Thyme, Red
Inner Strength

Botanical name	*Thymus vulgaris*
Note	top to middle
Method of extraction	steam distillation
Parts used	leaves and flowering tops
Fragrance	herbal, intense, medicinal, powerful, spicy
Color(s)	blue, red, yellow
Chakra(s)	heart, throat, third eye
Astrological sign(s)	Gemini
Planet(s)	Mercury
Number(s)	7
Animal(s)	elephant, hawk, whale
Element(s)	air

Affirmation I have great inner strength. I'm grounded, focused, and tuned in to the Universe. I stay on task with the projects at hand. I am always divinely protected. Even those situations that might initially appear to be negative are transformed to reveal the good.

Complementary flower essences *Elm* to overcome feelings of exhaustion, depression, and inadequacy. *Gorse* to improve faith to know that you will feel strong and happy again. *Rock Water* for strength and inner harmony. *Sweet Chestnut* to release exhaustion and darkness, replacing it with inner strength and light.

Complementary stones Amazonite, amethyst, blue calcite, blue lace agate, carnelian, copper, galena, green moss agate, emerald, tabular quartz, turquoise.

About the plant Thyme is a fragrant plant that reaches a height of about 1 foot. It has small leaves and pink or pale purple flowers.

Chemical components Thujanol, myrcenol, linalool, myrcene, caryophyllene, terpinen, myrtenyl acetate, terpineol, limonene, terpinene, pinene, sabinene, ocimenone.

Spiritual uses Use thyme to call upon Archangel Haniel to improve determination and to assist you in aligning with your soul's purpose. Thyme fortifies and increases courage, helping you to live your life in alignment with your true soul's agreements. It helps you remember who you truly are and encourages you to live this life to your fullest potential. It wards off psychic energy that may try to interfere with your highest purpose. Add it to blends to deflect and remove negative forces from your energy field and physical space. Use it to stay focused on your spiritual path and your personal spiritual truth. Thyme's vibration also facilitates telepathic communication. This essential oil assists in remembering the pure teachings of Atlantis.

Mental uses Thyme improves your memory and concentration. It clears your mind and literally activates brain cells to allow a clear flow of mental awareness and focus. Employ thyme to stay focused and on task so that you can more easily integrate the material into your consciousness, making it readily available when you need to retrieve it.

Emotional uses Add thyme to a synergistic blend when you feel emotionally exhausted. It helps you to release emotional blocks and feelings that bring your spirits down. It is useful to fight off symptoms of depression. This strong oil fortifies your inner strength, prompting you to overcome feelings of vulnerability and empower yourself.

Physical uses Thyme's most beneficial attribute is its ability to ward off infection. Use thyme as part of a synergistic blend for sore throats like tonsillitis and laryngitis as well as bronchitis. It is effective for reducing the symptoms of asthma. It prevents the spread of germs. It raises low blood pressure. Thyme is a good aromatherapy ally for chefs, dental professionals, dermatologists, ear/nose/throat specialists, housekeepers, infectious disease specialists, manicurists, mothers, nurses, and pulmonary specialists.

Therapeutic properties Analgesic, antibacterial, antibiotic, antidepressant, antifungal, anti-inflammatory, antimicrobial, antioxidant, antiparasitic, antipruritic, antiputrid, antirheumatic, antiseptic, antispasmodic, antitoxic, antitussive, antivenomous, antiviral, aperitive, aphrodisiac, astringent, balsamic, bronchodilator, cardiac, carminative, cicatrizant, counterirritant, cytophylactic, diaphoretic, digestive, diuretic, emmenagogic, febrifugal, hypertensor, insecticidal, nervine, rubefacient, sedative, stimulative, stomachic, sudorific, tonic, uplifting, warming.

Divine guidance Do you remember who you truly are? Are you searching for strength to deal with all that is going on in your life? Know that you are strong enough to overcome any challenge that arises throughout your life. Remember that you are always safe and have great inner strength.

For your safety Prolonged use may have a toxic effect. Possible skin irritant. Keep away from mucuous membranes and private parts. Avoid in cases of high blood pressure. Do not use if pregnant or nursing.

Interesting tidbits:
The use of thyme was prevalent throughout ancient Egypt, Greece, and Rome. Ancient Egyptians used it in the embalming process, and due to its germicidal properties, it was one of the oils purported to be beneficial during the plague in Europe. It was traditionally given to jousting knights for courage during the Age of Chivalry. Thyme was not originally used as a culinary herb but instead was burned for its smoke.

VETIVER
Tranquility and Peace

BOTANICAL NAME	*Vetiveria zizanioides*
NOTE	base
METHOD OF EXTRACTION	steam distillation
PARTS USED	roots
FRAGRANCE	musky, earthy
COLOR(S)	brown, dark blue, green, yellow
CHAKRA(S)	root
ASTROLOGICAL SIGN(S)	Capricorn, Taurus
PLANET(S)	Ceres, Earth, Saturn, Venus
NUMBER(S)	4, 44
ANIMAL(S)	earthworm
ELEMENT(S)	earth

Affirmation All is well. I am calm, relaxed, and at peace. I am grounded, focused, and energized. I have plenty of energy and time to accomplish what I need and want to get done. I live a spiritual, peaceful life. I spend quality time in nature every day. I have an intimate connection with Mother Nature and her loving tools for natural healing.

Complementary flower essences Clematis to maintain focus on the present moment. *Oak* to allow yourself time to rest and renew. *Rock Water* for balance and flexibility.

Complementary stones Brown agate, gold tiger's eye, hematite, sodalite, sugilite, tiger iron, tree agate, pyrite.

About the plant Vetiver is a tropical grass that reaches a height of up to 8 feet. It has sharp-edged leaves, small flowers, and aromatic roots.

Chemical components Khusimol, vetiselinenol, cyclocopacamphan, cadinol, vetivone, vetivenene, eudesmol, khusenic acid, vetispirene, amorphene, eudesm, calacorene, cadinene, ziza, selinene, eudesma, salvia, khusinol, selina, cubenol, eremophila, calacorene, prekhusenic acid, isovalencenol, spirovetiva, preziza, intermedeol, isokhusenic acid, elemol, juniper camphor, khusimone, funebran.

Spiritual uses Vetiver is a perfect essential oil for connecting with the elemental spirits, devic forces, and the fairy kingdom. It will also help you stay grounded during spiritual practices when used in very small amounts. This is a perfect oil for earth-centered spiritual pursuit, earth-based rituals, and shamanic journeywork. Vetiver helps to cleanse the auric field. Use this oil to align your energy with Archangel Raphael for grounding and healing and with Archangel Thuriel to amplify your connection with nature.

Mental uses Vetiver can be a useful tool for grounding. It is a good companion when you are trying to remain focused on your personal goals. Vetiver amplifies your ability to gather knowledge and wisdom from the universal consciousness. It helps you keep your thoughts aligned with your personal truth. It also helps you to more readily access the vast information stored within your own mind. Vetiver is calming and helps to relieve stress and tension.

Emotional uses Vetiver encourages you to take yourself into nature to rebalance raw emotions, feelings, and out-of-control responses. It calms your emotions and nerves while uplifting your mood to feel more aligned and balanced. Vetiver helps you master emotions during periods of emotional upheaval. According to Worwood in *The Fragrant Mind*, vetiver is a good tool to heal addiction to drugs, burnout, hysteria, grief, obsession, rage, repression, and stress.

Physical uses Vetiver encourages deep, restful sleep and helps relieve exhaustion. It also helps balance the reproductive system. Add this oil to a synergistic blend for the purpose of firmly establishing your body in the present moment with your feet connected to Mother Earth through your deeply embedded roots. It is a fixative for perfumes and stabilizes the volatile nature of essential oil blends. Vetiver loosens tight muscles and relieves pain. It is an insect repellent. It can also improve digestion. Vetiver is a good aromatherapy ally for architects, aromatherapists, cardiologists, contractors, ecologists, gardeners, herbalists, landscape architects, and librarians.

Therapeutic properties Abortifacient, analgesic, antibacterial, anti-inflammatory, antiparasitic, antiseptic, antispasmodic, antistress, aphrodisiac, astringent, calmative, cardiotonic, carminative, detoxifier, diaphoretic, diuretic, emetic, emmenagogic, insecticidal, nervine, revitalizing, rubefacient, sedative, stimulative (immune system), stomachic, tonic.

Divine guidance Is a situation in your life inflamed? Steps to reduce emotional, physical, and mental inflammation are in order. Try visualization and meditation to bring a new calmness to every aspect of your life and body. Peace and tranquility are yours for the asking. Connect with the image of firmly planted roots. Remember you have the ability to flex and bend in a storm—mentally, physically, spiritually, and emotionally. Allow the experiences of life to help you realize amazing growth. Remember your roots; yet always remember how much you can grow to reach great heights.

For your safety No known contraindications.

> **Interesting tidbits:**
> Vetiver grass has been hung in clumps over windows or placed within mattresses to ward off mosquitos.

WINTERGREEN
Attitude Adjustment

BOTANICAL NAME	*Gaultheria procumbens*
NOTE	middle
METHOD OF EXTRACTION	steam distillation
PARTS USED	leaves
FRAGRANCE	medicinal, penetrating, strong
COLOR(S)	green, white
CHAKRA(S)	all
ASTROLOGICAL SIGN(S)	Capricorn
PLANET(S)	Saturn
NUMBER(S)	13/4
ANIMAL(S)	dove, goat, rabbit
ELEMENT(S)	earth

Affirmation My physical structure is strong; all parts of my body feel good. My spine, bones, tendons, and muscles are healthy, strong, and aligned. I adjust my attitude to create a happier life for myself. I am discerning about the people I allow into my inner circle.

Complementary flower essences Chestnut Bud to recognize life patterns. *Sweet Chestnut* for strength. *White Chestnut* to release repetitive thoughts.

Complementary stones Ametrine, azurite, azurite-malachite, bloodstone, carnelian, chrysocolla, copper, elestial quartz, hematite, kyanite, lapis lazuli, orange calcite, purple-dyed agate, selenite, sodalite.

About the plant Wintergreen is a North American plant that reaches a height of about 6 inches. It has shiny deep-green leaves and white flowers that turn into red berries.

Chemical components Methyl salicylate.

Spiritual uses Wintergreen assists in releasing patterns of family and personal karma at a spiritual level. Use it to help you relax and release during spiritual healing sessions and regression therapy. In a synergistic blend, wintergreen adds healing energy to clear energetic blocks that have accumulated in the body. As you inhale wintergreen, call upon Saint Germain and Archangel Zadkiel for transformation and Archangel Raphael for healing.

Mental uses Wintergreen helps you release repetitive negative thoughts, mental conflict, and misperceptions by clearing your mind. The green energy of wintergreen envelops mental wounds and negative patterns like a healing salve.

Emotional uses Wintergreen's energetic signature is to remove pain. Add a drop of this oil to a synergistic blend to heal old emotional wounds. This oil gives you a boost when you need to figure out what emotions are buried in your subconscious mind. If you need to "uninstall" an emotional program, wintergreen's energy can help you gain a greater perspective by becoming the observer.

Physical uses Wintergreen relieves inflammation, pain, and all types of aches, including some of the symptoms of arthritis and rheumatism. Wintergreen is warming and improves circulation. Include wintergreen in a synergistic blend for sore and aching muscles. It is a great addition to revive your feet after long periods of standing. It promotes restful sleep and lowers blood pressure. Wintergreen is a good aromatherapy ally for chiropractors, dentists, doctors, marathon participants, physical therapists, Pilates instructors, runners, physical trainers, and Reiki practitioners.

Therapeutic properties Analgesic, antibacterial, anti-inflammatory, antirheumatic, antiseptic, antispasmodic, antitussive, astringent, carminative, decongestant, diuretic, emmenagogic, galactagogic, hemostatic, hypotensor, rubefacient, stimulative, tonic, vulnerary.

Divine guidance Do you need to take some time to seek spiritual fulfillment? Have you been experiencing physical inflammation? Are you experiencing physical aches? It is time to take care of yourself physically, spiritually, mentally, and emotionally. Take the time to balance your physical, mental, emotional, and spiritual energy.

For your safety Toxic in high doses. Inhibits blood clotting, so avoid use if on anticoagulants or undergoing surgery. Avoid in cases of low blood pressure. Possible skin irritant. Do not use if pregnant or nursing.

> **Interesting tidbits:**
> The main constituent in wintergreen is similar to salicylic acid in aspirin. Wintergreen is used to flavor many brands of toothpaste and chewing gum. It is one of the ingredients in root beer, along with sassafras and other natural flavors.

YLANG-YLANG
Love and Spiritual Affluence

BOTANICAL NAME	*Cananga odorata*
NOTE	base to middle
METHOD OF EXTRACTION	steam distillation
PARTS USED	flowers
FRAGRANCE	intense, floral, narcotic, sweet
COLOR(S)	pink, yellow, white
CHAKRA(S)	solar plexus, navel
ASTROLOGICAL SIGN(S)	Cancer, Libra, Pisces, Scorpio
PLANET(S)	Jupiter, Moon, Neptune, Venus
NUMBER(S)	8
ANIMAL(S)	dove
ELEMENT(S)	water

Affirmation All I need is always within reach. I am grateful for everything I have. Extraordinary love and amazing wealth on all levels are always available to me. I have an abundance of spiritual helpers ready to assist me in all areas of my life. The time is now!

Complementary flower essences Gorse to help you believe that life will get better and better every day.

Complementary stones Citrine, hematite, kunzite, lapis lazuli, malachite, morganite, rose quartz, ruby.

About the plant Ylang-ylang is a tropical tree that reaches a height of up to 100 feet. It has large yellow flowers that become black fruit with black seeds.

Chemical components Linalool, benzyl benzoate, germacrene, caryophyllene, geranyl acetate, methyl salicylate, cresol methyl ether, benzyl acetate, farnesyl acetate, methyl benzoate, cadinene, benzyl salicylate, geraniol, cadinol, muurolol, cinnamyl acetate, copaene, muurolene.

Spiritual uses Ylang-ylang encourages spiritual service to others. Employ this oil to help you recognize the abundance of spiritual helpers—master teachers, loved ones on the Other Side, saints, angels, goddesses, muses, and so on—available to you at all times. Use this oil to appeal to your guardian angels and Kuan Yin (the goddess of mercy and compassion) to guide you and instill spiritual wisdom within you. It is beneficial for meditation as it relaxes the chatter in your mind.

Mental uses Ylang-ylang relaxes the mind and relieves the internal dialogue that cycles through your consciousness. Ylang-ylang improves alertness and attentiveness. It aids in seeing love, feeling love, being love, and encouraging loving thoughts for yourself and others.

Emotional uses Use ylang-ylang to help calm erratic emotions; be mindful, though, as it brings feelings to the surface to allow for discussion and self-awareness. This oil helps you work through those feelings and relieve the pain of emotional blocks. Ylang-ylang helps relieve symptoms associated with depression, improves self-esteem, and encourages states of euphoria. It is a good oil for self-nurturing and helps you feel beautiful. When using ylang-ylang, imagine you are wrapped in a healing blanket of flowers filled with loving vibrations.

Physical uses Ylang-ylang is an aphrodisiac and is beneficial in fertility blends. Because of its stress-reducing properties, it lowers blood pressure, helps to improve sleep patterns, and reduces feelings of being overwhelmed. Ylang-ylang has some pain-reducing qualities, but overall it is a calming and relaxing oil. It encourages wealth and prosperity. Ylang-ylang is a good aromatherapy ally for cardiologists, hairstylists, insomnia specialists, counselors, doulas, marriage counselors, maternity nurses, meditation facilitators/practitioners, and sex therapists.

Therapeutic properties Antidepressant, antipruritic, antiseptic, aphrodisiac, calmative, carminative, emmenagogic, emollient, euphoriant, fixative, hypotensor, moisturizer, nervine, rejuvenator (skin and hair), relaxant, sedative, stimulative (circulatory system), tonic.

Divine guidance Are you ready to attract the best of everything? Do you believe the best is yet to come? Make a clear decision to manifest the good now in this moment. Don't wait until tomorrow. You are being called to experience spirituality in everyday living. See all the love that is in everything.

For your safety Avoid use in cases of low blood pressure. Do not use if pregnant or nursing.

Interesting tidbits:
Ylang-ylang has been referred to as "perfume tree." The name actually means "flower of flowers" in Tagalog (a Philippine language). The flowers have been used on the marriage beds of newlyweds for perfume and blessings. According to Rhind in her book *Fragrance and Wellbeing*, this oil provides the green top notes of Chanel's *No. 19* and Dior's *Miss Dior*.

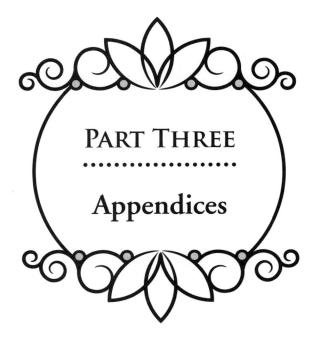

PART THREE

Appendices

Appendix A:
Aromatherapy Recipes For Specific Uses

Over the years, I've taught many classes on aromatherapy. Everyone's favorite part of the class is the time spent concocting formulas based on the goals and intentions of the participant. To start this process, it is important to establish why you want to create the blend, while keeping in mind which scents you prefer. As you have read throughout the book, there are many oils that can assist with the same type of issue or intention. Establish your goals on each level—spiritual, mental, emotional, and physical. Be sure to take note of any contraindications of a given essential oil; there are many choices, so there is no need to use one that might not be appropriate for your particular health condition.

You will need to have good quality bottles and caps (1 dram, 5 ml, and/ or 10 ml), pipettes, and the chosen essential oils on hand (see below). Be sure to purchase true medical grade oils, which I personally use. Then, take the following steps:

1. Establish your goal for the blend on all levels—physically, spiritually, mentally, and emotionally.

2. Determine which oils meet the needs of your goals on all four levels. Choose from three to ten oils.

3. Keep a pad handy to jot down which oils you will be using.

4. Using your pipette, place a few drops of the first oil into the bottle. Pause to smell the blend before adding the next oil. Adjust the scent by using more or less of a certain oil.

5. Keep a note of how many drops you use for each oil so you can re-create the blend at another time if you wish.

6. When your blend is complete, write the name of your blend on a sticky label and affix it to the bottle.

———

Below are sample recipes developed in various classes over the years, which I consider potent body, mind, and spirit formulas. The quantities given reflect how many drops to use. Feel free to adjust the recipes according to your needs and chosen oils, if desired.

Caregiver Formula

Bergamot to maintain mental clarity and good focus.............................8

Frankincense to align with the spiritual
  nature of the person being cared for...30

Orange for joy and encouragement...34

Ylang-ylang to maintain calm and inner peace......................................3

Vetiver to encourage focus and to stabilize the aroma............................2

Stress Reduction and Muscular Discomfort Relief

Bergamot to amplify self-confidence and raise self-esteem 18

Chamomile to release stress and encourage peaceful sleep....................... 1

Geranium to induce a sense of peace 4

Lemongrass to relieve muscular pain 13

Lavender to calm and relax.. 45

Patchouli to improve self-worth and strengthen the emotional body 3

Better Meditation Experiences

Cedarwood to clear negative thoughts and deepen spiritual practice..... 12

Chamomile to establish a sense of connection with guides and angels 2

Eucalyptus to encourage the use of
the breath and to clear energetic space.. 3

Frankincense (the ultimate oil for meditation)
to bring about mystical experiences.. 21

Lavender to experience tranquility and inner peace 60

Patchouli to evoke sudden flashes of enlightenment or awakening....... 3.5

Sage to release negativity and external negative influences..................... 12

Integrate Mind, Body, Spirit at Work

Grapefruit to sharpen memory and
mental clarity while aligning with angels.. 60

Rosemary to awaken your spiritual consciousness,
improve memory, and be in the present moment 12

Sage for safety from harm and divine protection.................................... 20

Sweet marjoram to maintain a sense
of calm during harrowing experiences 20

Radical Change and New Employment

Lemon to maintain a positive outlook and high self-confidence 60

Lime to encourage sweetness and provide cleansing and purification 40

Chill Out

Sacred Space

Sleep Well, Stay Positive

Clean the Floor

(Add 5 drops of this blend to 16 ounces of water and mop as usual. Use with caution and sparingly on wood floors as it might affect the finish over time.)

Lemon for its antifungal, antibiotic, antiparasitic, antiseptic
(strong), and disinfectant properties; refreshing, uplifting 10

Peppermint for its antibacterial, antibiotic,
antiseptic, antiviral, and insecticidal properties..................................5

Pine for its antibacterial, antifungal, antiparasitic, antiseptic (strong),
antiviral, deodorizer, and insecticidal properties; refreshing............... 20

Clean the House

(Use 3–5 of the oils listed to create a master blend. Add 5 drops of this blend to 16 ounces of water in a spray bottle.)

Clove for its antibacterial, antibiotic, antifungal, antiseptic
(strong), antiparasitic, antiviral, and insecticidal properties 1

Lemon for its antifungal, antibiotic, antiparasitic, antiseptic
(strong), and disinfectant properties; refreshing, uplifting 10

Niaouli for its antibacterial, antiparasitic,
antiseptic, and insecticidal properties 15

Orange for its antibacterial, antifungal, and antiviral properties..............5

Pine for its antibacterial, antifungal, antiparasitic, antiseptic (strong),
antiviral, deodorizer, and insecticidal properties; refreshing............... 20

Sage for its antibacterial, antifungal, antiviral,
disinfectant (strong), and insecticidal properties................................ 10

Tea tree for its antibacterial, antibiotic, antimicrobial,
antiparasitic, antiviral, and insecticidal properties; refreshing 5

Disinfectant for the Air and Body

Clove to disinfect the atmosphere of infectious disease 1

Eucalyptus to disinfect the atmosphere of infectious disease 25

Lavender to disinfect the atmosphere of infectious disease 45

Lemon to cleanse and detoxify, restore vitality, and release exhaustion......25

Ravensara to ward off germs that affect the respiratory
   system and to clear bacterial infections and viral attacks....................25

Tea tree to clear infections, fungus, germs, and viral conditions............25

Dust Mite Elimination

(Combine all ingredients in a spray bottle. Spray on bed daily. Wash linens
weekly in hot water.)

Eucalyptus radiata as an insecticide ....5 ml

Grain alcohol, 70 to 90 proof...1 oz

Rubbing alcohol ....3 oz

A few drops of your chosen blends can be added to Holy Water, Gemstone Essences, or plain distilled water to create energetic mists. Appendix C provides sample combinations of crystals for the creation of tinctures to heighten your intentions. Use the affirmations provided or create your own positive thoughts to match the blend and establish intention with each use. To add even more to the energetic component of your mist, add Bach Flower Essences as found in the Bach Flower Remedies Selection Guide in Appendix B. Holy Waters that you collect during your journeys and experiences in life also increase the vibration of peace, compassion, love, and well-being of your mist or blend. One drop of a Flower Essence, Gemstone Essence, or Holy Water will positively affect the energetic vibration of large and small quantities of blends.

Appendix B:
Bach Flower Remedies Selection Guide

Rescue Remedy® is the most widely known of the Bach Flower Remedies. It is a five flower formula that helps to prevent the disintegration of the energetic system while a person is going through trauma or severe stress. It is great to use while waiting for medical help in emergency situations. If you can't administer it in drinking water, moisten the lips with the remedy (all Bach Flower Remedies are intended to be taken by mouth). Whether you are dealing with bad news, fear, an accident, or any type of tragedy, this flower combination can help maintain the energetic integrity so self-healing can take place. Rescue Remedy can improve everyday life if you are in a stressful or traumatic profession, like an ER worker, and it can also alleviate everyday fears, like an impending visit to the dentist, an operation, or a divorce. It is also excellent for calming yourself or anyone in your care who has witnessed violence, whether on TV or in person.

The five flower formula includes Star of Bethlehem for trauma, Rock Rose for terror or panic, Impatiens for irritability, Cherry Plum for fear of losing control, and Clematis for staying present and connected.

While Rescue Remedy® is a great go-to formula, it is empowering and effective to discover and use a combination of flower essences specific to your personal mental and emotional challenges. Bach Flower Essences are divided into seven basic categories: fear, uncertainty, insufficient interest in present circumstances, loneliness, oversensitivity of influence and ideas, despondency and despair, and over-caring for the welfare of others. These categories make it easier to identify what you are feeling. You can ask yourself, "Do I feel apathy? Am I feeling oversensitive? Do I care for others too much and it is affecting my own well-being?" This type of categorization helps you sort through the thirty-eight Bach Flower Essences to find the one that will assist you in restoring balance.

Read through the descriptions of each of the essences within their larger categories and take note of which flower essences describe you the best. On a pad of paper, rate each category from 1–10, with 10 being the number that most closely describes your challenges. Then gift yourself with the vibrational healing experience by using these essences and watch them assist you in transforming your life.

Add the appropriate flower essence to your aromatherapy blend to create an aroma-energetic formula suited specifically to your needs. (After you add Bach Flower Essences to an essential oil blend, you can no longer take the essences internally.) The flower essence adds a vibrational element to the synergistic blend. The addition of the flower essences creates an aroma-energetic blend to spray on and around your body, which will help you effectuate change for the purposes intended energetically for the mental, emotional, and spiritual aspects of your consciousness.

Along with the descriptions of the remedy that follow, you will find an affirmation to use to support your transformation. Whenever you spray your aroma-energetic blend in your space or on and around your body, state the positive thought to affirm what you do want instead of focusing on the out-of-balance condition. Envision yourself restored and in alignment with your intended outcome.

Fear

Aspen is helpful for free floating anxiety and indefinable fear. It is beneficial for fear of the dark for all ages. Aspen is helpful for the elderly who are challenged by sundowners syndrome or unknown fear associated with dementia and Alzheimer's disease. (I saw the benefits of this remedy firsthand in my father when he was experiencing symptoms of senility.)

Ask yourself: Do you feel apprehension but don't know why? Do you have feelings of anxiousness and dread, but you can't put your finger on the source?

Aspen Affirmation: I am safe and sound. All is well. I am supported in all areas of my life. Everything is okay!

Cherry Plum comes to your assistance when you feel that you are going to "crack" or when the burdens of life are so intense or traumatic that you might even think you are going to have a nervous breakdown. This flower essence is helpful if you think you might hurt yourself or others. It is helpful for those suffering from irrational thoughts or mental illness. Note: If these symptoms persist, seek professional therapy.

Ask yourself: Do you feel out of control mentally, emotionally, or physically? Do you think about hurting yourself or someone else?

Cherry Plum Affirmation: I am composed. I am calm and collected. I breathe deeply and know that everything is under control.

Mimulus is perfect to use when you are worried and fearful about things you are aware of, whether it is worry about an upcoming event or a fear of public speaking. This is for those who are worried about the small things and also have challenges expressing their concerns and fears. Mimulus is a great aid to those who get tongue-tied when they need to speak or share their fears. It is helpful for those who perceive they have throat chakra challenges. (See the section on chakras in chapter 2.)

Ask yourself: Are you consciously experiencing fear—you know what you are afraid of—such as death, the dentist, heights, public appearances, tests, and other everyday life situations? Are you very shy or timid? Do you feel you are highly sensitive?

Mimulus Affirmation: I am safe. It is easy for me to interact with others. I am confident and courageous. Speaking in front of others is comfortable. I help others when I speak. I am always Divinely protected.

Red Chestnut is an excellent essence to use if you are obsessed with the care of another person. This is typically the type of care that is based on being overly concerned and fear that something dreadful will happen to your loved one. Sometimes the anticipation of something bad happening is not specific but more general. For example, a parent may be worried that something terrible will happen to his or her child. (This flower essence helped me release worries as a caregiver of my elderly parents.)

Ask yourself: Do you find yourself worrying about your loved ones? Is your mind preoccupied with concern over their well-being? Do you feel stress thinking that something bad will happen to those you care for?

Red Chestnut Affirmation: I am at peace. My mind is calm and relaxed. I am sure my loved ones are safe and sound.

Rock Rose is used for extreme fear or terror in a real life situation. It can be helpful if you feel your life is in danger. Use it after a horrific nightmare that leaves you shaken and perhaps even sweating. Rock Rose is one of the Bach Flower Remedies that can help you deal with post-traumatic stress disorder when you have "frozen" fears that render you unable to think or react.

Ask yourself: Are you frozen with fear? Do you fear for your life? Are you suffering from nightmares? Do you experience panic attacks?

Rock Rose Affirmation: I have the power to control my surroundings. I have the strength and coping skills to move through challenges. I am relaxed and confident. It is safe for me to be powerful in loving ways.

Uncertainty

Cerato is a good remedy to use for those who just can't make decisions and have a tendency to want to ask everyone else's advice. This essence is helpful for those who might be addicted to psychics or who have a tendency to ask the same question over and over again to intuitives even when they've received the same answers time and again.

Ask yourself: Do you look to others for advice and confirmation because you don't trust your own decision-making skills? Do you often question decisions you've made? Do you go back and forth, changing direction because your self-confidence is lacking?

Cerato Affirmation: I know my own truth and trust the wisdom from within myself. I look within and know the answers. I trust my own intuition and gut feelings.

Gentian restores hope and confidence. It is a great aid for those who give up easily because of a minor setback. They are creative with great ideas yet have challenges bringing the ideas to fruition. They might have the best intentions and goals for the future but often find excuses or allow a diversion to keep them from fulfilling their goal.

Ask yourself: Have you observed that you have a negative attitude that stops you from taking action to complete something? Are you easily discouraged or get down in the dumps if things go wrong? Do you disengage from a project at the slightest delay or challenge?

Gentian Affirmation: I have courage and confidence. I can achieve anything I put my mind to. It is easy for me to resolve challenges as they arise. I am motivated and enthusiastic.

Gorse is for those who have heavy, dark energy around them because they have a strong sense of hopelessness and despair. They believe that life will never get any better. They often feel like it is not worth the trouble to overcome their challenges and that there is no point in trying. Gorse is helpful for those suffering from an illness when they have no faith that any treatment will be successful. They are very pessimistic.

Ask yourself: Do you believe that you can overcome any challenge? Have you given up all hope? Do you perceive that there is absolutely nothing that can be done to overcome your pain or trials and tribulations?

Gorse Affirmation: There is always help and there is always hope. Life is just a cycle and these challenges will pass soon. I envision myself healthy, happy, and peaceful. I know that every day I get better and better in every way!

Hornbeam is perfect to use when you are feeling overwhelmed and exhausted before you even start your day or the project. Use it when your tendency is to procrastinate, not because you are too tired but more because you just don't feel like it. The vibration association is the Monday morning blues. This is a remedy that helps you get started and motivated so you can recognize that the project or task at hand isn't so bad at all!

Ask yourself: Do you have the tendency to put off tasks that are simple to complete? Can you accomplish things you enjoy but feel too tired or overwhelmed to handle chores or responsibilities that aren't as enjoyable? Do you procrastinate because you don't feel like doing some things that you can and do easily complete?

Hornbeam Affirmation: I am full of energy and enthusiasm. I am motivated and feel satisfied by all my accomplishments daily. I am a productive person. I enjoy everything I do!

Scleranthus is helpful if your timing is off and you therefore miss opportunities. Mood swings and unreliability are often the cause of uncertainty and indecisiveness. This is a good remedy for those who have a hard time making a decision about anything. Whether it is a big or small decision, there is vacillation and trouble deciding even the small things like what to eat or what to wear.

Ask yourself: Are you nervous? Do you have a tendency to be fidgety? Have you observed that you are moody? Do you vacillate when making decisions regardless of their importance?

Scleranthus Affirmation: I am always at the right place at the right time. I trust my own inner knowing. It is easy for me to make decisions.

Wild Oat is the perfect remedy for someone who is still trying to figure out what to do with his or her life. It is for those who feel like they have a special purpose but can't put their finger on what it is. The perfect career or life path seems to elude them. This remedy is also for those who spend a lot of time wondering what to do and avoid responsibilities because they prefer to loaf around or hang out using this excuse of not knowing what to do with their life.

Ask yourself: Do you believe you have a block that prevents you from fulfilling unknown dreams? Are you always searching for the right job or life path to bring you joy?

Wild Oat Affirmation: I receive guidance and inspiration all the time. I am grateful for my right livelihood. I am blessed to do what I love. I am clear on my life path.

Loneliness

Heather flower essence is helpful to those who are overly talkative and obsessed with their own life and/or troubles. This is the type of person who doesn't give you a chance to speak during a conversation. They are usually alone or lonely and often avoided because they aren't very good listeners and can be draining to be around.

Ask yourself: Do you allow others to share their experiences during conversations? When you've spent time with another person, can you recall if you gave them a chance to talk about their life? Are you a good listener or do you prefer to do all the talking?

Heather Affirmation: I am very interested in the well-being of my friends and family. I listen well. It is easy for me to stay focused on others as they speak and really hear what they are saying. I am balanced in my conversational abilities.

Impatiens is of great assistance to those who are impatient with people who are foolish or slow. It also helps increase tolerance with coworkers who might not be as fast as you are at performing tasks. It's good for those who are intelligent yet have little patience for those who don't catch on to things as quickly as they do. It is helpful if you have a tendency to get bored by non-stimulating or uninteresting conversation. This remedy is good if you have a tendency to speak, act, and think quickly.

Ask yourself: Are you short-tempered with people who are slower than you in body or mind? Would you rather work alone? Do you feel that you must always rush to get through things?

Impatiens Affirmation: There is plenty of time to get things done. I am grateful for my coworkers. I am patient, kind, and tolerant. I am relaxed and enjoy life. I take the time to observe the beauty in nature and my surroundings.

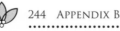

Water Violet is helpful for those who are quiet and prefer to be alone or with just a few friends. This remedy is helpful if you have a tendency to be proud or distant. If you have a tendency to feel you are superior to others, then water violet can aid in bringing balance to foster a connection with others. This remedy is good for developing trust and humbleness.

Ask yourself: Do others perceive you as full of yourself and unfriendly? Are you withdrawn and do you prefer to be alone without distractions from others?

Water Violet Affirmation: I am aligned with this present moment. I interact well with my friends and family. It is easy for me to relate to and trust others. I am actively involved in the lives of friends.

Insufficient Interest in Present Circumstances

Chestnut Bud is helpful for people who keep making the same mistakes in life over and over again. This remedy helps those who don't realize they are repeating the same mistake by allowing the same types of circumstances to evolve. In other words, the names and faces may have changed, but the same issue keeps occurring, and they still haven't learned the lesson. This remedy can help you recognize negative patterns and the answer to "Why is this happening to me?"

Ask yourself: Are you making the same mistakes time and again? Does it take you a while to realize you choose the wrong friends or partners or jobs? Are you recognizing your mistakes and learning from them?

Chestnut Bud Affirmation: I learn from my experiences. I find great value in the lessons learned from my mistakes and failures, and I use those lessons to create success! It is easy for me to recognize life patterns and use them to make future decisions.

Clematis flower essence is a remedy for those who escape reality and the present moment. It is helpful for those who are absentminded and withdraw from interaction with society. This type of person is someone who isn't happy with his or her present circumstance but doesn't really do anything about changing it. This is a good remedy to use if you are unable to stay focused and feel a bit spacey.

Ask yourself: Do you have a hard time staying focused for any length of time? Are you preoccupied and not present in most life circumstances? Do you feel out of it?

Clematis Affirmation: I am grounded and focused. It is easy for me to stay present and fully engaged in the moment. I am truly aligned and connected with my circle of family and friends.

Honeysuckle is beneficial for those who live in the past and don't have expectations for much happiness in the future. It's helpful when you find yourself a bit too nostalgic and wanting things to be like they used to be instead of embracing what is occurring in this time of your life.

Ask yourself: Is your focus on the past and the way things used to be? Are you reminiscing a bit too much over a time gone by, a past success, or a lost love? Is your nostalgia preventing you from living fully present in this moment?

Honeysuckle Affirmation: I am grateful for the wonderful friends and family in my life. My future is filled with happiness. I enjoy my life every day and every moment!

Mustard is for those who have a tendency to feel gloomy or depressed. Mustard is helpful if you feel like there is always a dark cloud or negative vibes following you around even if you don't know the reason why you feel this way.

Ask yourself: Do you feel like you have a dark cloud over your life? Do you find yourself suddenly depressed? Do you tend to be unhappy?

Mustard Affirmation: I am filled with lightness and joy. I am happy, whole, and complete. I find pleasure and delight in even the small blessings in my life. I love to smile and laugh!

Olive is a remedy I have found helpful for caregivers who are physically and mentally exhausted to the point that they just don't have any more to give. It is beneficial to help to accept rest and recognize that daily life doesn't have to be so hard. This remedy helps you reconnect with life's pleasures.

Ask yourself: Do you feel like everything takes a monumental effort? Are you exhausted because of a long period of anxiety and stress?

Olive Affirmation: I take the time I need to rest and rejuvenate. I am strong and have plenty of energy. Every day in every way my body, mind, and spirit regenerate and find balance.

White Chestnut is perfect to help you release the incessant chatter in your mind. Use White Chestnut when you have worrisome thoughts that prevent you from being able to work or feel peace.

Ask yourself: Are you unable to sleep because your thoughts are keeping you awake? Are you lacking mental peace? Have you been worried about things that aren't likely to occur? Do you have repetitive thoughts that circle around in your consciousness, and you can't seem to get them to stop?

White Chestnut Affirmation: My mind is clear. My emotions are calm. I am at peace. I have a quiet mind.

Wild Rose is for those who are apathetic and find an interest in nothing. This essence is helpful when you feel that your creative juices are low and you lack energy and enthusiasm for most things. It helps to release feelings of monotony and unhappily accepting life as it is.

Ask yourself: Are you resigned to accepting things as they are? Do you find life monotonous? Are you unhappy but not doing anything about it to bring more happiness?

Wild Rose Affirmation: I seek out and embrace the joys of living. I never give up and find ways to enjoy life. I am an optimist. I am looking forward to assisting others to bring more happiness.

Oversensitivity of Influence and Ideas

Agrimony is for those who will avoid an argument and agree to things even if it doesn't suit them. Use this if you are going through a period in your life when you have to make believe you are happy and all is well, even when you aren't happy. It is helpful to use if you are drawn to drugs or alcohol use to help you deal with the current life challenges.

Ask yourself: Do you hide your worries behind a smiling face to avoid revealing your pain or challenges? Will you have a drink or take drugs to help you cope with the pressures of life? Do you give in easily to others to avoid conflicts?

Agrimony Affirmation: I am relaxed, open, and honest. I am at peace. I attract people who are trustworthy. I easily share my problems, hopes, and wishes.

Centaury is best to use when you realize you are being of service to others at the expense of your own well-being. Centaury is good to use if you let people take advantage of your good nature. This is a helpful remedy if you want to change the fact that you always take on the role of helper rather than leader.

Ask yourself: Are you easily influenced by others who have stronger personalities than you? Do you feel timid and subservient? Do you have a hard time saying no? Do you let people impose upon your good nature?

Centaury Affirmation: I have a strong sense of self. I am courageous. It is easy for me to set boundaries in loving ways. I am firm and fair. It is safe for me to be powerful.

Holly can assist you when you are feeling insecure and jealous of others. It helps you realign when you feel angry and tend to be overly aggressive. This remedy can help if you have been emotionally hurt from a betrayal of a friend or after a relationship breakup. It is especially beneficial when you can't think clearly because of hurt feelings, which might cause you to be more suspicious or jealous.

Ask yourself: Are you harboring feelings of dislike and jealousy? Are you feeling anger toward others? Do you assume everyone has an ulterior motive?

Holly Affirmation: I attract trustworthy people. I am happy for the good fortune and blessings of others. I feel inner peace and calm. I am filled with love and compassion for others and myself. I am a loving, kind person. My words are spoken with love and kindness.

Walnut is helpful during times of change, like ending or starting a new relationship or moving to a new residence. It's helpful for life cycle transitions from puberty to menopause. Walnut can also help during career or job changes. It helps you break attachments or habits. Walnut is beneficial when changing from one way of being to another, such as healing addictions or mindsets.

Ask yourself: Are you going through changes physically, mentally, spiritually, or emotionally? Are you in the process of breaking a bad habit or addiction? Are you moving or changing jobs?

Walnut Affirmation: Events from my past have a positive effect on my present and future. My emotions are balanced. Even when the world around me is constantly changing, I remain grounded and focused.

I embrace change. I recognize that it can usher in improved life situations. I am grateful for the balanced flow of energy within me.

Despondency and Despair

Crab Apple is a good remedy when you are in the process of shedding weight or releasing habits that make you feel less than good about yourself. Use crab apple to help balance obsessive-compulsive behavior that is preventing you from dealing with more pressing life challenges. This flower essence is beneficial for relieving the feeling of being contaminated or infected or if you have tendencies toward overly high standards of cleanliness.

Ask yourself: Do you obsessively wash your hands or clean your surroundings and feel overly concerned about germs and infections? Are you embarrassed about your appearance and believe you aren't attractive? Have you been focusing on unimportant imperfections while avoiding more important issues?

Crab Apple Affirmation: I am healthy, whole, and complete. My body is perfect. I am the perfect weight for my height, build, and genetics. I stay focused on what is truly important. I know I am safe and sound.

Elm is the flower essence to turn to when you are overwhelmed. It is especially beneficial for successful people who typically excel in their work, are efficient, and hold a position of responsibility. Employ the vibration of this flower essence to help you through periods in which you are temporarily challenged by too much work, self-doubt, or temporary exhaustion and feelings of depression.

Ask yourself: Are you feeling overwhelmed by responsibility and work? Are you lacking confidence, feeling inadequate, and unable to deal with everything? Do you perceive that there are just too many tasks ahead of you?

Elm Affirmation: I have plenty of time for everything I need to do. I complete tasks fully. I stay focused on the present. My life flows naturally. I relax into everything I do and truly enjoy it.

Larch is for those who expect to fail, lack confidence, and have a tendency toward pessimism. Use this remedy during periods of life when you might feel inferior and fear failure. This essence is beneficial for those who know on some level, even secretly, that they have what it takes to do what they need to do. Employ the vibration of this flower essence when you notice that you are missing out on opportunities because of these fears, which you might perceive as a block.

Ask yourself: Do you believe that you have a block? Do you feel that you aren't good enough and are often disheartened? Are you lacking self-esteem and feeling inferior to others? Are you missing opportunities?

Larch Affirmation: I am always in the right place at the right time. I have the courage and confidence to succeed. I do what it takes to achieve my goals and aspirations. There are plenty of people who recognize my good qualities. I see the good within myself. I allow others to see my inner sparkle.

Oak is for the type-A person who has exhausted themselves. This remedy is for a strong, reliable, and responsible person who has now worn themselves out but doesn't want anyone to perceive them as weak. They have a tendency to struggle on valiantly instead of admitting that they need to take time to renew.

Ask yourself: Are you relentless? Are you an overachiever? Do you hide the fact that you are exhausted and need time to care for your own needs? Are you exhausted but must continue on even though you are draining yourself physically, mentally, and emotionally?

Oak Affirmation: I enjoy relaxing in nature to regenerate and rejuvenate my energy field. It is safe for me to be vulnerable. I willingly nurture myself and others who truly need and want my nurturing. Today, I take steps toward caring for myself. I honor my body and my sacred space.

Pine is for someone who is always apologizing even if the fault doesn't lie with him or her. Use pine flower essence when you have a guilty conscience that is not based on reality. This remedy aids you if you have a tendency to take the blame for the mistakes of others. Use pine to help you release feelings of guilt and regain mental and emotional peace.

Ask yourself: Do you feel guilty? Are you taking the blame for anything that goes wrong even when it had nothing to do with you? Are you setting your goals so high that you set yourself up so you'll never be able to satisfy them?

Pine Affirmation: I am calm. I am at peace. I easily achieve my goals. I know that any intense feelings of guilt or self-blame will pass as I release them from my body. It is easy for me to embrace a happy life. I regenerate the love I have for myself.

Star of Bethlehem is for rebalancing after a shock. I have seen the benefits of using it after devastating tragedies such as the loss of a family member in a disaster. In fact, this remedy was in high demand during the aftermath of September 11. It is a helpful remedy for conditions that result from other types of shocking and extremely stressful events as well. While it is commonly used directly after a shock, this remedy also offers benefits in the case of post-traumatic symptoms arising years after the event. This is one of the essences included in Rescue Remedy.

Ask yourself: Have you experienced a sudden death, disappointment, or accident? Are you feeling numbed or experiencing a nervous breakdown?

Star of Bethlehem Affirmation: I am revitalized. I am safe and sound. All is well. Nurturing energy heals and balances me on all levels—mentally, physically, spiritually, and emotionally.

Sweet Chestnut is helpful when you are so distraught and distressed that nothing consoles you. It is useful to rebalance you during times when you feel that you have great despair and there is no hope. When you feel that you have reached the outer limits of your endurance, use Sweet Chestnut to release sorrow, suffering, exhaustion, loneliness, and darkness.

Ask yourself: Is your outlook on life bleak and dark? Are you feeling unbearable anguish? Do you feel you do not have strength or the endurance to carry on?

Sweet Chestnut Affirmation: I see the light at the end of the tunnel. I have a peaceful mind. My faith is strong and provides me with support. I have great inner strength.

Willow is for those periods of time when one is self-obsessed and experiencing self-pity. Use this if you are resentful and bitter. This flower essence is useful if you lack gratitude and are never pleased. You might feel jealous or angry because of other people's luck, health, success, and happiness. Use it when you are irritable and have a gloomy outlook.

Ask yourself: Do you find yourself saying things like "I don't deserve this" or "Why is this happening to me"? Have you been alienating friends and family because of your resentful attitude? Are you critical of others, especially those who are happy and healthy?

Willow Affirmation: I forgive and forget past injustices. I enjoy life and attract positive people and situations. I realize that my thoughts and emotions create my own circumstances. I am grateful for all the good in my life.

Over-caring for the Welfare of Others

Beech is helpful to increase your ability for tolerance and acceptance of others. Use this remedy when you are feeling superior to others and are being judgmental and arrogant. This flower essence aids you during times when you are easily agitated by other people's lifestyles or behaviors. This remedy is helpful if you are a perfectionist and feel you are always right.

Ask yourself: Do you often think that the way other people handle things is never done right? Do you believe your way is the right way and everyone else is wrong? Are you easily annoyed by the lifestyle or mannerisms of others?

Beech Affirmation: I live and let live. I see the good in others. I accept the imperfections we all have. I am tolerant and accepting.

Chicory can help you when you are controlling and have manipulating tendencies toward your loved ones. This remedy is for strong-willed people who are critical and overly demanding. Chicory can be of benefit when you are too mothering, smothering, or overprotective.

Ask yourself: Do you want others to conform to your beliefs and standards? Are you overprotective of your loved ones? Do you have expectations of others when you give your love and attention to them? Do you dislike being alone and want constant attention? Are you argumentative?

Chicory Affirmation: All my friends and family are safe and sound. They are Divinely protected. I am relaxed and know all is well. My loved ones—friends and family—have their own paths to travel, and I trust their innate abilities to traverse their lives. I allow others to live their own lives.

Rock Water is for those who set extremely high standards for themselves and work very hard and excessively to meet their own high standards. If you are fanatical about work, exercise, or any goal you have set for yourself, use this remedy to be more flexible and relaxed. This flower essence will help you integrate the truth that the power of inner strength is greater than extreme disciplines or forced behaviors.

Ask yourself: Are you overly opinionated? Are you overly self-focused but at the same time deny yourself relaxation to the point of becoming a self-inflicted martyr? Do you find yourself rigid in your determination to stay on course with diet, exercise, and other routines?

Rock Water Affirmation: I have balance in my life. It is easy for me to relax. It is safe for me to be vulnerable. I experience inner peace and harmony. I go with the flow.

Vervain is perfect during times of high tension and hyperactivity. This is an excellent balancing remedy to assist those who are extremely determined, hard-working, and over-achieving. Use this when you go beyond the limits of your abilities and your mind is racing. If you have a tendency to say yes to many projects, find it challenging to say no, and take on too many projects or jobs at once, use this remedy until you balance out your life.

Ask yourself: Is your plate full and you have still accepted more work and responsibility? Do you find yourself suffering from extreme muscle tension? Do you have an inability to relax? Is your over-the-top enthusiasm potentially alienating others?

Vervain Affirmation: I allow myself to just be. Great things are achieved in stillness. Sometimes taking no action is much more powerful than taking action. I am calm, wise, and tolerant. It is easy for me to relax.

Vine is for when you find that you are feeling bossy and domineering. This remedy helps to balance you when you have a tendency to bully others or put them down. You might be extremely gifted, intelligent, ambitious, and a natural leader, and this flower essence can assist to calm your aggressive nature that comes across as a lack of compassion or kindness. This rigidity might also manifest as high blood pressure. For those who are the boss or leader, this essence helps to temper the gifts you share so that they are received with more consideration and kindheartedness.

Ask yourself: Do you always take charge in projects, meetings, or conversations? Do you have the tendency to believe your way of doing things is the only right way to do things? Are you manipulative and do you enjoy your status of power and authority over others?

Vine Affirmation: I speak with kindness and compassion. I communicate what is on my mind in a gentle way. I speak eloquently and lovingly. I am accepting of others exactly as they are. I am generous with my time, and I am fully present with my friends, family, and colleagues.

Appendix C:
Gemstone Essences

In this appenedix you will find suggested combinations of gemstones for a specific intention. These are the gemstones I recommend for each intention. Gather these stones together to create a vibrational essence. Add the vibrational Gemstone Essence water to your aromatherapy blends to magnify the energetics and intentions for the given blend. Do not ingest Gemstone Essence water. Remember to start by establishing the purpose of the essence and place the stones into the water with focused intent. Use your own intuition and pick stones that you resonate with. Follow the instructions in the "How to Make a Gemstone Essence" section in chapter 2.

Love

Invoke Archangel Chamuel for healthy relationships and healing.

Blue Lace Agate—for ease in communication and to amplify recognition of angelic guidance.

Citrine—to activate self-confidence and to improve the ability to set boundaries.

Green Aventurine—to draw in good fortune and blessings.

Pink Calcite—to encourage happiness, harmony, comfort, and good companionship.

Rose Quartz—to attract romance, good friends, and love.

Unakite—to activate kindness, compassion, and balance.

Love Affirmation: I am love, and all that surrounds me and all that is attracted to me is love. I attract love, joy, and happiness into my life.

Protection

Invoke Archangel Michael for protection, faith, and removal of fears, phobias, and obsessions.

Amethyst—to activate the transformation of challenging situations.

Black Tourmaline—to deflect negativity and increase safety.

Clear Quartz—to amplify intentions of well-being and love.

Gold Tiger's Eye—to repel jealousy and bad intentions of others.

Snowflake Obsidian—to find the lesson and move on.

Sodalite—to amplify Archangel Michael's protective presence.

Protection Affirmation: All is well. I surround myself with trustworthy people. I am blessed, and I am always Divinely protected.

All Is Well

Invoke Archangel Uriel for wisdom, peace, and higher guidance.

Citrine—to amplify courage and confidence and to improve prosperity-consciousness.

Garnet—to ground your intentions, get motivated, and take action.

Green Aventurine—for good luck and good fortune and to increase the incoming flow of money.

Jade—to amplify the blessings of prosperity.

Pyrite—to create a strong foundation and do what you love.

Red Tiger's Eye—to stay focused on the goal and deflect negative distractions.

All Is Well Affirmation: I am blessed with abundance. I am fortunate, and I appreciate my prosperity. I am grateful for all my creative and business skills. I earn unlimited income doing what I love.

Develop Your Intuition

Invoke Archangel Gabriel for inspiration, psychic messages, and dream symbol interpretation.

Amethyst—to improve dreaming and psychic messages that come through dreams.

Angelite—to communicate, hear, and connect with angels, archangels, and master teachers.

Clear Quartz—for mental clarity and focus.

Moonstone—for greater perspective and to amplify receptivity and awareness of life cycles.

Selenite—to increase connection with higher consciousness and spirit guides.

Sodalite—to improve and encourage meditation, contemplation, and prayer.

Develop Your Intuition Affirmation: I am extremely intuitive. I receive Divine messages all the time. It is easy for me to interpret the messages and guidance I receive. I am profoundly clairvoyant.

Angel Communication

Invoke Archangel Michael to attract an entourage of angelic helpers and guardian angels.

Angelite—to communicate, hear, and connect with angels, archangels, and master teachers.

Blue Lace Agate—for Divine communication and alignment with soul's purpose.

Celestite—to reawaken your angelic self and connection with Divine timing.

Selenite—to increase connection to the Divine, your guardian angel, and your entourage of invisible helpers.

Seraphinite—to facilitate communication with the angelic realm.

Turquoise—to increase reception of the channel of Divine inspiration.

Angel Communication Affirmation: I am grateful for the angelic orchestration at play in my life. Angels are providing guidance to me all the time. I allow angels to work through me to provide healing for others and myself.

Sound Sleep

Invoke Archangel Sabrael to release negative thoughts and forces and to ward off incessant mind chatter.

Amethyst—to ward off nightmares and encourage sweet dreams and restful sleep.

Apatite—to help you focus on a healthy digestive system.

Green Aventurine—to recalibrate your emotions each night when kept near your heart.

Hematite—to remove scattered energy from your energy field and repel negative thoughts.

Rose Quartz—to align your consciousness with Divine love, compassion, mercy, tolerance, and kindness.

Purple-dyed Agate—to help you transform negative thoughts and believe in unlimited possibilities for the good.

Sound Sleep Affirmation: I take good care of myself by eating healthy foods and getting exercise. I sleep well every night. I am calm and peaceful. All is well, and life is good.

Creativity and Fertility

Invoke Archangel Haniel, the angel of Divine communication and Nature Spirits, Elementals, and Muses, to open up your channels of inspiration.

Carnelian—to give yourself the time to create and the courage to take the action to make it so.

Chrysocolla—for shamanic journeywork or engaging in deep meditative practices to tap into Divine inspiration.

Citrine—to activate the courage and confidence to live your life to your fullest potential.

Orange Calcite—to encourage action and play and to foster a fertile life.

Red Goldstone—to activate your imagination.

Turquoise—to know, speak, express, and live your truth.

Creativity and Fertility Affirmation: Creativity flows through me. I am courageous and bravely bring my ideas into actuality. My imagination is the key to my success. I envision my future and joyfully participate as it unfolds.

Aura Cleansing

Invoke St. Germain and Archangel Zadkiel for transformation, transmutation, and the Violet Flame. The Violet Flame is used by spiritual alchemists for self-transformation and elevation to higher spiritual truths.

Amethyst—for its powerful transformative qualities.

Chrysoprase—for encouragement to engage in nurturing practices.

Howlite—for cleansing and purification.

Kyanite—to align your energy centers with the higher realms.

Rose Quartz—to feel comforted and surrounded by unconditional love.

Selenite—to clear negative vibrations and replace them with light, love, and well-being.

Aura Cleansing Affirmation: Blessings flow through me like a healing river. I am fluid. I am pure and clear. My chakras are balanced. I am aligned with the Divine.

Perfect Weight and Healthy Eating

Invoke Archangel Camael to align with the Divine masculine and release anger, aggression, and negative emotions, and to have more movement and exercise.

Apatite—to become aware of emotional eating.

Chrysoprase—to have the courage and confidence for self-care.

Clear Quartz—to help you transmit and transduce energy.

Garnet—to improve energy levels and boost metabolism.

Howlite—for cleansing and to obtain higher understanding of the source of emotional stress.

Peridot—to support the digestive system and the optimal functioning of the gallbladder, liver, pancreas, and spleen.

Perfect Weight and Healthy Eating Affirmation: I am healthy, whole, and complete. My body is perfect. I am the perfect weight for my height, build, and genetics. I exercise regularly, drink plenty of water, sleep well, and eat healthy, nutritious foods.

Good Health and Healing

Invoke Archangel Ariel for general health and vitality.

Chrysoprase—to help rebalance and clear out overwhelming feelings.

Green Aventurine—to focus on eating healthy and regular exercise.

Garnet—to connect to the vital life force, blood flow, and the circulation of other fluids throughout the body, and the alignment of the spinal column.

Jade—to help with kidney ailments and general good health.

Peridot—for the proper assimilation of nutrients of food, drink, water, and light.

Rose Quartz—for regeneration and skin rejuvenation.

Good Health and Healing Affirmation: I am healthy, whole, and complete. My body is full of energy and vitality.

Keep Me Safe

Invoke Archangel Melchizedek to aid your spiritual journey on Earth.

Amethyst—to protect you from psychic attacks and clear out negative thoughts.

Black Obsidian—to keep you grounded and aligned with the truth.

Black Tourmaline—to deflect negative energy.

Hematite—to maintain a state of relaxed focus and to relieve stress.

Rose Quartz—to amplify love and well-being.

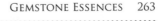

Selenite—to deflect negativity and increase love and well-being.

Keep Me Safe Affirmation: I am safe and sound. All is well. I am always Divinely protected.

Sobriety

Invoke Archangel Michael for protection, faith, and removal of fears, phobias, and obsessions.

Amethyst—to avoid harmful distractions and to change old habits through conscious intent.

Clear Quartz—for financial success, fertility, creativity, family blessings, happy home, and healthy body.

Hematite—to maintain a sense of calm.

Black Tourmaline—to understand the source of negative energy and triggers.

Rose Quartz—to connect your human existence as a grounded individual with your spiritual life purpose.

Green Aventurine—to amplify your belief in good fortune and well-being and to create a positive and stable reality for yourself.

Sobriety Affirmation: I am safe. I am blessed. It's easy for me to transform and transmute challenging situations.

Appendix D:
Easy Reference Guide to Associated Oils

This appendix provides you with an easy way to find the oils that are a vibrational match for archangels, Ascended Masters, astrological signs, asteroids, planets, careers, and professions. Use this section to get to know the energetic vibration of a given essential oil. This appendix makes it easy for you to make a synergistic blend and strengthen the intention associated with the formula.

Archangels and Ascended Masters
This section provides essential oil suggestions listed by archangel and Ascended Masters as a quick and easy way to look up a list of oils that could work to petition the help and energetic vibration of the angels.

Archangel Ariel (general health and vitality)—lemongrass

Archangel Auriel (realignment of the Divine Feminine and subconscious fears)—angelica, clary sage, jasmine, mandarin, neroli, sweet marjoram

Archangel Camael (realignment of the Divine Masculine, anger, aggression, and emotions)—celery seed, clary sage, grapefruit, spruce

Archangel Chamuel (relationship healing)—palmarosa, rose

Archangel Gabriel (inspiration and guidance, dream interpretation, and inner knowing)—angelica, bergamot, chamomile (Roman), lavender, mandarin, palmarosa, rose, tea tree

Archangel Haniel (Divine communication, determination, and alignment with soul's purpose)—palmarosa, rose, thyme

Archangel Jophiel (inner wisdom and beauty)—grapefruit, jasmine, neroli, sweet marjoram

Archangel Melchizedek (aiding the spiritual journey on Earth and connection with the mystic within)—bergamot

Archangel Metatron (activation of the ascension process to higher states of consciousness, enlightenment, Akashic records, and the soul's evolution)—basil, grapefruit, palmarosa, rose

Archangel Michael (protection, faith, and removal of fears, phobias, and obsessions)—allspice, angelica, basil, bergamot, black pepper, chamomile (German), eucalyptus, grapefruit, mandarin, sweet marjoram

Archangel Muriel (rebalancing of emotions)—neroli, peppermint

Archangel Raphael (healing for yourself and others)—benzoin, birch, elemi, geranium, jasmine, juniper berry, lavender, orange, oregano, tea tree, vetiver, wintergreen

Archangel Raziel (embracing the gifts of clairvoyance, prophecy, revelation, and the great mysteries)—angelica, black pepper

Archangel Sabrael (release of jealousy, viruses, and negative forces)—basil, celery seed, geranium, lavender, palo santo, rosemary

Archangel Thuriel (animal healing and human connection with nature)—vetiver

Archangel Tzaphkiel/Zaphkiel (the feminine aspect of God, understanding and mindfulness)—frankincense, spikenard

Archangel Uriel (thoughts, ideas, creativity, insight, alchemy, astrology, universal consciousness, Divine order, cosmic universal flow, Earth's environment, illumination, and peace)—chamomile (Roman), frankincense, orange, oregano, spikenard

Archangel Zadkiel (transformation, transmutation, and the Violet Flame)—wintergreen

Buddha—frankincense, sandalwood

Christ—frankincense, myrrh, spikenard, spruce

Guardian Angel (one's main guardian)—angelica, mandarin, niaouli, orange, rose, ylang-ylang

Isis—myrrh, spikenard

Kuan Yin—jasmine, lavender, neroli, orange, rose, sandalwood, spikenard, ylang-ylang

Mary Magdalene—myrrh, spikenard

Mother Mary—jasmine, myrrh, neroli, rose, spikenard

Our Lady of Guadalupe—rose

Pallas Athene—bergamot, ginger

Saint Germain—angelica, benzoin, grapefruit, hyacinth, lavender, wintergreen

Saint Therese of Lisieux—jasmine

Astrological Signs

This section provides essential oil suggestions listed by astrological sign as a quick and easy way to look up a list of oils that could work to align with the astrological qualities of the astrological vibration.

Aries—anise seed, black pepper, celery seed, clove, eucalyptus, lilac, mandarin, orange

Taurus—benzoin, German chamomile, lemon, melissa, sweet marjoram, rose, vetiver

Cancer—anise seed, bergamot, cardamom, celery seed, clary sage, coriander, elemi, fennel, geranium, ginger, lemon, myrrh, oregano, palmarosa, peppermint, rose, ylang-ylang

Gemini—birch, clove, eucalyptus, fennel, grapefruit, lemon, oregano, spruce, thyme

Leo—allspice, anise seed, basil, bergamot, cinnamon, grapefruit, lavender, lemon, lemongrass, lime, mandarin, niaouli, orange, petitgrain, rosewood

Virgo—anise seed, cardamom, coriander, fennel, German chamomile, ginger, grapefruit, lavender, lime, niaouli, rose, rosemary, spikenard

Libra—birch, black pepper, cedarwood, cinnamon, helichrysum, hyacinth, jasmine, juniper berry, lavender, mandarin, myrrh, neroli, palmarosa, ravensara, rose, sweet marjoram, ylang-ylang

Scorpio—anise seed, benzoin, blue cypress, geranium, helichrysum, hyssop, jasmine, lemongrass, neroli, niaouli, palo santo, peppermint, ravensara, sage, sweet marjoram, ylang-ylang

Sagittarius—cinnamon, clove, orange, petitgrain, pine, rosewood, spruce

Capricorn—allspice, birch, cedarwood, celery seed, coriander, hyacinth, lavender, neroli, pine, vetiver, wintergreen

Aquarius—angelica, birch, elemi, frankincense, hyacinth, lavender, mandarin, patchouli, sandalwood, spinkenard, tea tree

Pisces—angelica, bergamot, chamomile, clary sage, frankincense, hyacinth, juniper berry, oregano, patchouli, peppermint, sandalwood, spikenard, ylang-ylang

Asteroids and Planets

This section provides essential oil suggestions listed by asteroids and planets as a quick and easy way to look up a list of oils that could work to align with the astrological qualities of the asteroid or planet

Ceres—blue cypress, coriander, sweet marjoram, vetiver

Chiron—blue cypress, chamomile, hyssop, lavender, peppermint

Earth—cedarwood, fennel, lavender, niaouli, pine, vetiver

Juno—ginger, jasmine, neroli, spikenard

Jupiter—angelica, anise seed, cinnamon, clove, geranium, juniper berry, petitgrain, pine, rosewood, sweet marjoram, ylang-ylang

Mars—black pepper, celery seed, clove, eucalyptus, hyssop, orange, peppermint, rosemary, spruce

Mercury—birch, cinnamon, clove, coriander, eucalyptus, fennel, ginger, grapefruit, lemon, oregano, rosemary, spruce, sweet marjoram, thyme

Moon—anise seed, bergamot, cardamom, clary sage, coriander, elemi, fennel, geranium, ginger, jasmine, lavender, myrrh, neroli, oregano, palmarosa, peppermint, sage, wintergreen, ylang-ylang

Neptune—angelica, anise seed, bergamot, chamomile, clary sage, hyacinth, juniper berry, oregano, sandalwood, spikenard, ylang-ylang

Pallas Athene—bergamot, ginger

Pluto—benzoin, blue cypress, celery seed, helichrysum, hyacinth, hyssop, jasmine, neroli, niaouli, palo santo, peppermint, ravensara, rose, sage

Saturn—allspice, benzoin, birch, cedarwood, celery seed, coriander, vetiver, wintergreen

Sun—allspice, anise seed, basil, bergamot, chamomile, cinnamon, grapefruit, lavender, lemon, lemongrass, lime, mandarin, niaouli, orange, petitigrain, rosewood

Uranus—angelica, elemi, frankincense, mandarin, patchouli, rosemary, sandalwood, spikenard, tea tree

Venus—birch, chamomile, cinnamon, frankincense, geranium, helichrysum, hyacinth, jasmine, juniper berry, lemon, mandarin, melissa, myrrh, neroli, palmarosa, ravensara, rose, spikenard, vetiver, ylang-ylang

Careers and Professions

This section provides essential oil suggestions listed by careers and professions as a quick and easy way to look up a list of oils that could work to petition the help and energy of the oil to help you achieve your full potential. The oils are allies for these walks of life.

Accountant—grapefruit, lemon, lime, niaouli, rosemary

Actor—black pepper, ginger

Acupuncturist—frankincense, spikenard

Angel Communicator—grapefruit, jasmine, mandarin, melissa, rose, spikenard

Arborists—cedarwood, coriander, patchouli, pine

Architect—vetiver

Aromatherapist—benzoin, coriander, grapefruit, vetiver, spikenard

Artist—black pepper, blue cypress, cinnamon, hyssop

Astrologer—elemi

Athlete—birch, eucalyptus, German chamomile, sweet marjoram

Author—bergamot, blue cypress, German chamomile, grapefruit

Baker—anise, allspice, cinnamon, clove, mandarin

Banker—basil, lemon, lime, rosewood

Beekeeper—benzoin, blue cypress, melissa, rose

Body worker—birch, clove, spikenard

Broker—basil, rosewood

Builder—rosewood

Cardiologist—coriander, rose, spikenard, sweet marjoram, vetiver, ylang-ylang

Caregiver—birch, lime, melissa, myrrh, niaouli, ravensara

Chef—anise, lime, oregano, rosemary, sage, thyme

Chiropractor—spikenard, wintergreen

Clairvoyant—elemi, German chamomile, hyacinth, rose, sage, spikenard

Conservationist—juniper berry, melissa, pine

Contractor—benzoin, vetiver

Counselor—benzoin, bergamot, cardamom, palmarosa, rosewood, sage, sweet marjoram, ylang-ylang

Dental professional—birch, clove, geranium, myrrh, niaouli, oregano, peppermint, ravensara, tea tree, thyme, wintergreen

Dermatologist—cedarwood, rose, tea tree, thyme

Dietician—bergamot, cardamom, fennel, grapefruit

Doctor—wintergreen

Doula—clary sage, fennel, geranium, helichrysum, jasmine, sage, ylang-ylang

Drug rehabilitation specialist—bergamot, clary sage, elemi, helichrysum, jasmine, juniper berry, sweet marjoram

Ear/nose/throat specialist—clove, eucalyptus, frankincense, lime, niaouli, oregano, ravensara, rosemary, spruce, sweet marjoram, tea tree, thyme

Ecologist—cedarwood, pine, vetiver

Editor—bergamot, grapefruit, lime

Engineer—cardamom

Entrepreneur—basil, cinnamon, mandarin

Environmentalist—black pepper, cedarwood, clove, eucalyptus, lemongrass, peppermint, rosemary, rosewood

Esthetician—helichrysum, rose

Farmer—juniper berry, pine

Feng shui practitioner—clove, mandarin, orange, palo santo, sweet marjoram

Fertility specialist—clary sage, ginger, jasmine, neroli

Finance Manager—basil

Florist—juniper berry, pine

Gardener—coriander, juniper berry, patchouli, pine, vetiver

Gastroenterologist—bergamot, cardamom, celery seed, fennel, Roman chamomile, palmarosa

Ghost hunter—benzoin, cedarwood, palo santo, sage, sweet marjoram

Graphic designer—black pepper, blue cypress, cinnamon, clove, hyssop, peppermint

Grief counselor—hyacinth, jasmine

Gynecologist—clary sage, fennel, geranium, jasmine, neroli, sage

Hairstylist—cedarwood, rosemary, spikenard, ylang-ylang

Healthcare practitioner—birch, frankincense, juniper berry, lemon, ravensara

Heart surgeon—coriander, spikenard, vetiver

Herbalist—ginger, vetiver

Hospice caregiver—benzoin, birch, clary sage, grapefruit, helichrysum, hyacinth, melissa, myrrh, spikenard

Housekeeper—cedarwood, eucalyptus, lavender, lemon, niaouli, orange, pine, ravensara, spruce, tea tree, thyme

Infectious disease specialist—cedarwood, eucalyptus, lavender, lemon, niaouli, orange, pine, ravensara, tea tree, thyme

Insomnia specialist—lavender, spikenard, sweet marjoram, ylang-ylang

Intuitive reader—angelica, bergamot, cardamom, elemi, frankincense, German chamomile, grapefruit, palo santo, sage, spikenard

Inventor—blue cypress, celery seed, cinnamon, Roman chamomile, rosewood

Judge—bergamot, cardamom, hyssop, myrrh, sage

Keynote speaker—frankincense

Landscape architect—cedarwood, coriander, juniper berry, patchouli, pine, vetiver

Law enforcement professional—allspice, anise seed, basil, benzoin, cedarwood, clove, eucalyptus, geranium, hyssop, myrrh, pine, rosemary, sage, sweet marjoram

Lawyer—bergamot, lemon, myrrh, petitgrain, spikenard, sweet marjoram, tea tree

Leader—basil, bergamot, cinnamon, ginger, grapefruit, lemon

Librarian—benzoin, rosemary, sage, spikenard, spruce, vetiver

Life coach—frankincense, niaouli, palmarosa, petitgrain, rosewood, spruce

Manicurist—lime, niaouli, ravensara, tea tree, thyme

Marathon participant—birch, eucalyptus, sweet marjoram, wintergreen

Marriage counselor—basil, clary sage, coriander, geranium, ginger, jasmine, rose, rosemary, rosewood, sweet marjoram, ylang-ylang

Massage therapist—geranium, grapefruit, lavender, petitgrain

Maternity nurse—jasmine, ylang-ylang

Mediator—benzoin

Meditation facilitator/practitioner—angelica, bergamot, cedarwood, clary sage, elemi, frankincense, German chamomile, palmarosa, petitgrain, sage, sandalwood, ylang-ylang

Medium—myrrh

Mental health counselor—angelica, clary sage, jasmine, lime, mandarin, palmarosa, petitgrain, spruce

Merchant—basil, cinnamon

Metaphysician—angelica

Minister—cedarwood, frankincense, helichrysum, sage

Mother—anise seed, geranium, neroli, orange, rose, spikenard, tea tree, thyme

Musician—angelica, black pepper, blue cypress, cardamom, celery seed, cinnamon, lavender, mandarin, neroli, petitgrain, sage

Mystic—angelica, bergamot, black pepper, frankincense, ginger, hyacinth, jasmine, neroli, sandalwood, spikenard, spruce

Neurologist—allspice, angelica, bergamot, cedarwood, chamomile (German and Roman), elemi, grapefruit, orange, oregano, palmarosa, patchouli, peppermint, petitgrain, rosemary, sage, spikenard

New age retailer—frankincense, lavender, myrrh, sage, sandalwood

Nurse—birch, niaouli, ravensara, tea tree, thyme

Nutritionist—grapefruit

Parent—lavender, mandarin, neroli, orange, spikenard

Pest control professional—black pepper, clove, eucalyptus, lemongrass, peppermint, rosemary, rosewood

Phlebotomist—basil, geranium, sage

Physical therapist—birch, German chamomile, wintergreen

Physical trainer—birch, clove, German chamomile, wintergreen

Pilates instructor—clove, wintergreen

Pilot—lemon

Podiatrist—niaouli, ravensara, tea tree

Psychologist—rosewood, sage

Publisher—bergamot, black pepper, blue cypress, grapefruit, lime

Pulmonary specialist—eucalyptus, frankincense, hyssop, palo santo, peppermint, ravensara, spruce, sweet marjoram, tea tree, thyme

Regression therapist—basil, clove, peppermint

Reiki practitioner—birch, frankincense, lavender, sage, wintergreen

Runner—wintergreen

Sex therapist—clary sage, ginger, hyacinth, jasmine, patchouli, rose, sandalwood, ylang-ylang

Shamanic practitioner—birch, cedarwood, chamomile (Roman), palo santo, ravensara, sage, spruce

Speaker—angelica, chamomile (Roman), tea tree

Spiritual counselor—birch, frankincense, helichrysum, hyacinth, sage

Spiritual healer—birch, sage

Teacher—benzoin, chamomile (German)

Travel professional—ginger, lavender, sweet marjoram

Vascular doctor—oregano

Veterinarian—petitgrain

Visionary leader—sandalwood, spikenard, spruce

Wedding planner—orange, rose, rosemary, rosewood, sweet marjoram

Weight-loss/weight-gain counselor—celery seed, grapefruit

Writer—black pepper, blue cypress

Yoga practitioner/instructor—patchouli

Chakras

This section provides essential oil suggestions listed by chakra as a quick and easy way to look up a list of oils that could work for a given chakra.

Crown—allspice, angelica, benzoin, bergamot, black pepper, cardamom, clove, eucalyptus, frankincense, grapefruit, helichrysum, hyacinth, hyssop, jasmine, juniper berry, lavender, myrrh, neroli, orange, palo santo, peppermint, ravensara, rosemary, sandalwood, spikenard, spruce, sweet marjoram, wintergreen

Third eye—allspice, angelica, anise seed, basil, birch, black pepper, chamomile (German), cinnamon, clary sage, clove, eucalyptus, frankincense, hyacinth, juniper berry, lavender, lime, palo santo, peppermint, rosemary, spruce, sweet marjoram, tea tree, thyme, wintergreen

Throat—allspice, angelica, clove, eucalyptus, chamomile (German), lavender, oregano, niaouli, palo santo, peppermint, ravensara, sandalwood, sweet marjoram, tea tree, thyme, wintergreen

Heart—allspice, anise seed, cedarwood, chamomile (Roman), elemi, eucalyptus, frankincense, ginger, grapefruit, helichrysum, hyacinth, jasmine, lavender, lime, mandarin, neroli, orange, oregano, palo santo, palmarosa, patchouli, peppermint, petitgrain, rose, rosewood, sandalwood, spikenard, spruce, sweet marjoram, tea tree, thyme, wintergreen

Solar plexus—allspice, anise seed, bergamot, blue cypress, cardamom, cedarwood, celery seed, chamomile (Roman), cinnamon, clary sage, clove, coriander, elemi, eucalyptus, fennel, ginger, grapefruit, helichrysum, lavender, lemon, lemongrass, lime, mandarin, melissa, niaouli, orange, oregano, palo santo, palmarosa, patchouli, peppermint, petitgrain, rosewood, sage, sandalwood, wintergreen, ylang-ylang

Navel—allspice, anise seed, basil, blue cypress, celery seed, cinnamon, clary sage, clove, coriander, elemi, eucalyptus, geranium, ginger, juniper berry, lavender, lemongrass, mandarin, melissa, niaouli, palo santo, palmarosa, peppermint, ravensara, sage, sandalwood, sweet marjoram, wintergreen, ylang-ylang

Root—allspice, basil, benzoin, black pepper, blue cypress, cedarwood, eucalyptus, ginger, hyssop, lavender, melissa, myrrh, niaouli, palo santo, patchouli, peppermint, pine, ravensara, sage, sandalwood, spikenard, vetiver, wintergreen

Physical, Mental/Emotional, and Spiritual Uses

This section provides essential oil suggestions listed by condition as a quick and easy way to look up a list of oils that could work for a given condition. I recommend you refer to the individual profiles to read more about the suggested oils. The listing is divided into three sections: physical, mental/emotional, and spiritual. The italicized oils are the most effective for the use indicated.

Physical Uses

Acne—birch, cedarwood, *chamomile (German)*, *lavender*, lemongrass, petitgrain, *tea tree*

Addiction—jasmine, *juniper berry*

Allergies—blue cypress, *eucalyptus*, *niaouli*, *ravensara*, *sweet marjoram*

Aphrodisiac—black pepper, ginger, hyacinth, jasmine, juniper berry, *neroli*, palmarosa, *patchouli*, *peppermint*, rosemary, rosewood, sandalwood, thyme, vetiver, *ylang-ylang*

Appetite (balance)—cardamom, celery seed, *lemon*, palmarosa

Appetite (increase)—*cinnamon*, mandarin

Arthritis/rheumatism—angelica, *birch*, blue cypress, cedarwood, *celery seed*, cinnamon, coriander, frankincense, *wintergreen*

Asthma—angelica, anise seed, eucalyptus, hyssop, *frankincense*, niaouli, pine, ravensara, spruce, *sweet marjoram*, thyme

Athlete's foot—palmarosa, *tea tree*

Bacterial infection—angelica, basil, benzoin, black pepper, blue cypress, cinnamon, *clove*, coriander, elemi, *eucalyptus*, fennel, *frankincense*, geranium, ginger, grapefruit, hyssop, jasmine, lavender, lemon, lemongrass, melissa, neroli, *niaouli*, *orange*, *oregano*, palmarosa, patchouli, peppermint, pine, *ravensara*, rosemary, rosewood, sandalwood, spikenard, *sweet marjoram*, *tea tree*, *thyme*, vetiver, wintergreen

Bites and stings (insect)—allspice, anise seed, blue cypress, *eucalyptus*, geranium, *lavender*, oregano, patchouli, *peppermint*, sweet marjoram, *tea tree*

Blood pressure (increase)—birch, *eucalyptus*, hyssop, geranium, orange, peppermint, pine, *rosemary*, *sage*, *thyme*

Blood pressure (reduce)—angelica, black pepper, cardamom, cedarwood, celery seed, chamomile, clary sage, lavender, lemon, lemongrass, melissa, neroli, rose, sweet marjoram, wintergreen, ylang-ylang

Body odor/deodorizer—benzoin, bergamot, coriander, eucalyptus, geranium, lavender, *lemongrass*, myrrh, neroli, patchouli, *petitgrain*, pine, *rosewood*, sandalwood, spikenard

Boils—bergamot, *chamomile (German)*, *lavender*, ravensara

Breathing and respiratory relief—*eucalyptus*, fennel, *frankincense*, peppermint, *ravensara*, *sweet marjoram*, wintergreen

Bronchitis—angelica, anise seed, eucalyptus, *frankincense*, hyssop, lime, *niaouli*, oregano, *pine*, *sweet marjoram*, thyme

Burns—*lavender*, niaouli

Children, fear—lavender, melissa, *orange*

Chills/chilliness/cold hands and feet—allspice, black pepper, clary sage, *cinnamon*, clove, coriander, *ginger*, frankincense, oregano, rosemary, *sage*, spruce, sweet marjoram, thyme, *wintergreen*

Circulation (poor)—benzoin, birch, *black pepper*, *cinnamon*, geranium, lemongrass, mandarin, niaouli, *oregano*, wintergreen

Colds—*eucalyptus*, frankincense, niaouli, *ravensara*, *sweet marjoram*, tea tree

Cold sores—*eucalyptus*, geranium, *ravensara*, tea tree

Constipation/healthy bowel movement—*anise seed*, basil, benzoin, bergamot, birch, black pepper, chamomile, coriander, *fennel*, ginger, hyssop, lemon, orange, oregano, patchouli, peppermint, pine, rosemary, sage, *spikenard*, sweet marjoram

Coughs—black pepper, *eucalyptus*, fennel, *frankincense*, peppermint, *ravensara*, *sweet marjoram*, thyme, wintergreen

Cramps—see muscle spasms

Cuts—see wounds

Digestion—allspice, angelica, *anise*, basil, bergamot, cardamom, *celery seed*, *cinnamon*, clary sage, coriander, fennel, ginger, grapefruit, juniper berry, *lemon*, mandarin, melissa, orange, palmarosa, patchouli, pepper, *peppermint*, petitgrain, rosemary, sage, spikenard, sweet marjoram, thyme

Earache—*chamomile (German)*, *eucalyptus*, lavender

Fertility—anise, *clary sage*, *geranium*, ginger, hyacinth, jasmine, juniper berry, neroli, palmarosa, patchouli, pepper, peppermint, sage, ylang-ylang

Fever reduction—angelica, basil, bergamot, birch, black pepper, cinnamon, coriander, *eucalyptus*, ginger, hyssop, lemon, *lemongrass*, lime, melissa, niaouli, orange, oregano, palmarosa, patchouli, peppermint, ravensara, *sage*, sandalwood, spikenard, *sweet marjoram*, thyme

Fungal infections—angelica, chamomile, clove, elemi, *eucalyptus*, fennel, geranium, juniper berry, lavender, lemongrass, myrrh, neroli, *niaouli*, orange, *oregano*, palmarosa, patchouli, pine, rosemary, rosewood, sage, sandalwood, spikenard, sweet marjoram, *tea tree*, *thyme*

Gout—*birch*, black pepper, blue cypress, cedarwood, *celery seed*, wintergreen

Gum infections—*clove*, *myrrh*, niaouli, peppermint, sage, *tea tree*

Headache—angelica, anise seed, *clary sage*, eucalyptus, ginger, *lavender*, lemongrass, *peppermint, sweet marjoram*

Heartburn and indigestion—anise, fennel, *chamomile*

Herpes zoster (shingles)—bergamot, *eucalyptus radiata*, geranium, *lavender, melissa, ravensara*

Impotence—*jasmine, neroli*, patchouli, *ylang-ylang*

Inflammation—angelica, benzoin, *birch*, blue cypress, cardamom, *chamomile (German and Roman)*, cinnamon, *clary sage*, clove, coriander, *eucalyptus*, fennel, frankincense, geranium, ginger, hyssop, jasmine, juniper berry, *lavender*, melissa, myrrh, orange, oregano, palo santo, patchouli, peppermint, rose, sage, sandalwood, *spikenard*, spruce, tea tree, thyme, vetiver, *wintergreen*

Insecticide—basil, benzoin, bergamot, birch, black pepper, blue cypress, *cedarwood*, cinnamon, clove, *eucalyptus radiata*, fennel, geranium, juniper berry, lemon, *lemongrass*, lime, melissa, palo santo, *patchouli*, peppermint, pine, rosemary, rosewood, sage, sandalwood, tea tree, thyme, vetiver

Insect repellent—blue cypress, eucalyptus, geranium, lemongrass, palo santo, *patchouli*, vetiver

Insomnia and restful sleep—*chamomile (German and Roman)*, coriander, clary sage, elemi, lavender, jasmine, mandarin, melissa, myrrh, neroli, petitgrain, orange, spikenard, sweet marjoram, vetiver, ylang-ylang

Jet lag—black pepper, *eucalyptus*, lemongrass, grapefruit, *lemon*, lime, mandarin, niaouli, *peppermint*, *rosemary*, spruce, tea tree

Joint aches and pain—allspice, *birch*, blue cypress, *celery seed*, *chamomile*, coriander, *lemongrass*

Lice—patchouli, *rosemary*, *tea tree*, ylang-ylang

Memory—*basil*, black pepper, coriander, ginger, grapefruit, *lemon*, melissa, *rosemary*, thyme

Menopause—*chamomile*, *clary sage*, fennel, *geranium*, ginger, jasmine, *lavender*, sage, *spikenard*

Menstrual problems—*chamomile* (German and Roman), *clary sage*, fennel, *geranium*, ginger, hyssop, jasmine, *lavender*, *melissa*, *neroli*, palmarosa, sage

Mental clarity and focus—black pepper, eucalyptus, grapefruit, lemongrass, *lemon*, lime, mandarin, niaouli, *peppermint*, *rosemary*

Migraine—clary sage, eucalyptus, *lavender*, *sweet marjoram*

Motion sickness—ginger, *peppermint*

Muscle aches and relaxant—bergamot, *birch*, blue cypress, *cedarwood*, clove, eucalyptus, lavender, *lemongrass*, neroli, orange, petitgrain, pine, *spikenard, sweet marjoram, vetiver, wintergreen*

Muscle spasms—neroli, petitgrain, *spikenard, sweet marjoram*, vetiver

Nail fungus—angelica, *chamomile (German and Roman)*, clove, elemi, eucalyptus, fennel, geranium, juniper berry, lavender, lemongrass, myrrh, neroli, niaouli, orange, *oregano*, palmarosa, patchouli, pine, rosemary, *tea tree, thyme*

Pain relief—allspice, angelica, anise seed, basil, bergamot, *birch*, black pepper, blue cypress, celery seed, *chamomile (German and Roman)*, cinnamon, *clary sage, clove*, coriander, elemi, *eucalyptus*, frankincense, geranium, ginger, jasmine, juniper berry, *lavender, lemongrass*, melissa, myrrh, neroli, niaouli, oregano, palmarosa, palo santo, patchouli, *peppermint*, pine, ravensara, rosemary, rosewood, sandalwood, *spikenard, sweet marjoram*, tea tree, thyme, vetiver, *wintergreen*

Parasites—benzoin, bergamot, birch, cardamom, *chamomile (German and Roman)*, cinnamon, *clove, eucalyptus*, fennel, geranium, ginger, hyssop, juniper berry, lavender, lemon, melissa, niaouli, *oregano*, palmarosa, patchouli, peppermint, pine, rosemary, rosewood, sage, spikenard, tea tree, thyme, vetiver

Perspiration (decrease)—*clary sage*, elemi, lemongrass, *sage*

Perspiration (increase) diaphoretic—angelica, *birch, black pepper*, celery seed, chamomile, coriander, eucalyptus, fennel, *ginger*, hyssop, lemon, melissa, *niaouli*, oregano, patchouli, sweet marjoram, *rosemary*, sandalwood, spruce

Pneumonia—*eucalyptus*, benzoin, *frankincense*, niaouli, *ravensara*, sweet marjoram

PMS—*chamomile, clary sage*, fennel, geranium, ginger, jasmine, lavender, sage

Respiratory problems—anise seed, benzoin, *eucalyptus*, *frankincense*, ginger, lavender, lime, *niaouli*, oregano, pine, ravensara, *spruce*

Sedative—benzoin, bergamot, black pepper, blue cypress, cedarwood, celery seed, *chamomile (German and Roman)*, *clary sage*, frankincense, *geranium*, hyacinth, jasmine, juniper berry, *lavender*, lemon, lemongrass, *mandarin*, *melissa*, *myrrh*, neroli, orange, patchouli, *petitgrain*, ravensara, sandalwood, *spikenard*, spruce, *sweet marjoram*, thyme, vetiver, ylang-ylang

Seduction/sex—allspice, anise seed, benzoin, cardamom, celery seed, cinnamon, *clary sage*, clove, coriander, geranium, ginger, hyacinth, jasmine, juniper berry, neroli, palmarosa, *patchouli*, pepper, peppermint, rosemary, sage, sandalwood, thyme, vetiver, *ylang-ylang*

Sinus congestion—*eucalyptus*, *frankincense*, hyssop, lavender, niaouli, pine, *ravensara*, *spruce*, *sweet marjoram*, *tea tree*

Skin care—benzoin, cedarwood, clary sage, *eucalyptus*, frankincense, *geranium*, grapefruit, jasmine, *lavender*, lemongrass, *myrrh*, neroli, niaouli, palmarosa, patchouli, *pine, rose*, rosemary, rosewood, ylang-ylang

Sunburn—*lavender*, niaouli

Throat aches and pain—*clove*, lime, *niaouli*, oregano, ravensara, rosemary, rosewood, sandalwood, spruce, sweet marjoram, *tea tree*, thyme

Toothache/dental infections—clove, niaouli, tea tree, wintergreen

Warts—clove, *eucalyptus*, cypress, elemi, lavender, lime, melissa, orange, *oregano*, palmarosa, patchouli, peppermint, pine, ravensara, rosemary, *tea tree*

Wounds—bergamot, elemi, *lavender*, melissa, myrrh, orange, *tea tree*

MENTAL/EMOTIONAL USES

Anxiety/calming—benzoin, bergamot, black pepper, blue cypress, cedarwood, celery seed, *chamomile (German and Roman)*, *clary sage*, frankincense, *geranium*, hyacinth, jasmine, juniper berry, *lavender*, lemon, lemongrass, *mandarin*, *melissa*, *myrrh*, neroli, orange, patchouli, *petitgrain*, ravensara, sandalwood, *spikenard*, spruce, sweet marjoram, thyme, vetiver, ylang-ylang

Blues/depression (relief of symptoms)—*bergamot*, celery seed, clove, frankincense, *geranium*, jasmine, lavender, *lemon*, lime, melissa, *palmarosa*, *petitgrain*, rose, *rosewood*, *sage*, thyme, ylang-ylang

Career/entrepreneurial success—*basil*, black pepper, *cinnamon*, clove, mandarin, rosemary

Clarity—allspice, anise seed, basil, benzoin, *bergamot*, birch, cardamom, black pepper, clove, coriander, *frankincense*, ginger, *grapefruit*, lavender, *lemon*, lemongrass, *lime*, mandarin, niaouli, palo santo, peppermint, *rosemary*, rosewood, spruce

Confidence—anise seed, basil, *bergamot*, black pepper, chamomile (German and Roman), cinnamon, clove, ginger, grapefruit, jasmine, juniper berry, *lemon*, lemongrass, lime, melissa, neroli, *orange*, *palmarosa*, patchouli, *petitgrain*, *rosewood*, sandalwood, sweet marjoram

Confusion—*basil*, benzoin, *bergamot*, birch, blue cypress, cardamom, *frankincense*, grapefruit, *lemon*, *lime*, myrrh, *palo santo*, *rosemary*, sage

Courage—angelica, anise seed, basil, *bergamot*, black pepper, celery seed, cinnamon, clary sage, *clove*, fennel, ginger, grapefruit, hyacinth, jasmine, *lemon*, neroli, orange, *petitgrain*, rose, rosewood, sweet marjoram, thyme

Fear—bergamot, *clary sage*, elemi, grapefruit, jasmine, lime, mandarin, neroli, orange, *palo santo*, rosemary, sage, *sweet marjoram*

Focus/grounding—allspice, anise seed, basil, benzoin, bergamot, black pepper, *cedarwood*, coriander, *frankincense*, geranium, grapefruit, juniper berry, lemon, lime, myrrh, niaouli, orange, palo santo, *patchouli*, peppermint, pine, ravensara, *rosemary*, thyme, vetiver

Friendship—allspice, blue cypress, geranium, *lemongrass*, neroli, rose, *rosemary*, sweet marjoram

Hysteria/rampant emotions—*clary sage*, frankincense, lavender, myrrh, *spikenard, sweet marjoram*

Joy/happiness—*bergamot*, chamomile, clary sage, *grapefruit*, jasmine, *lemon*, lemongrass, lime, mandarin, neroli, *orange*, patchouli, petitgrain, rose, rosewood, spruce, sweet marjoram

Law of attraction—*cinnamon, clove*, jasmine, juniper berry, mandarin, orange, *petitgrain*, ravensara, rose, ylang-ylang

Memory—*basil*, black pepper, clove, coriander, ginger, grapefruit, *melissa*, neroli, *rosemary*, thyme

Money/abundance—allspice, *basil*, black pepper, cinnamon, clove, mandarin, *orange, patchouli*, petitgrain, rosemary, rosewood, *spruce, ylang-ylang*

Nervousness/nervous exhaustion—angelica, basil, celery seed, *chamomile, clary sage*, coriander, elemi, *frankincense*, hyssop, juniper berry, lavender, lemongrass, *melissa*, orange, palmarosa, patchouli, peppermint, petitgrain, rosemary, sage, sandalwood, *spikenard*, spruce, *sweet marjoram*, thyme, *vetitver*

Nightmares—anise seed, *mandarin*

Positive attitude—*allspice*, anise seed, benzoin, *bergamot*, cardamom, cedarwood, clove, elemi, *grapefruit*, hyacinth, jasmine, juniper berry, lavender, *lemon*, mandarin, neroli, orange, palmarosa, *petitgrain*, rosemary, sage, sandalwood, *spruce*, sweet marjoram

Protection/"Keep Me Safe"—allspice, anise seed, *basil, benzoin, cedarwood*, chamomile, *clove*, eucalyptus, *geranium*, hyssop, myrrh, palmarosa, *palo santo, pine, rosemary, sage, sweet marjoram*, thyme

Romance—ginger, jasmine, orange, palmarosa, patchouli, *petitgrain*, rose, rosemary, *rosewood*, sandalwood, *sweet marjoram*, *ylang-ylang*

Safety—allspice, anise seed, basil, *benzoin, cedarwood*, clove, eucalyptus, geranium, hyssop, myrrh, rosemary, sage, *sweet marjoram*

Shock/trauma—hyacinth, lavender, myrrh, *sweet marjoram*, tea tree

Sorrow/grief—*blue cypress, hyacinth*, hyssop, jasmine, neroli, myrrh, palo santo, patchouli, rose

Stress—allspice, anise seed, basil, benzoin, bergamot, cedarwood, chamomile, *clary sage*, clove, fennel, geranium, grapefruit, hyacinth, jasmine, juniper berry, *lavender, lemongrass*, mandarin, melissa, neroli, *orange*, palmarosa, palo santo, patchouli, petitgrain, rosewood, sandalwood, spikenard, spruce, *sweet marjoram*, vetiver, ylang-ylang

Study/memory—*basil*, lemon, lime, *rosemary*

Worry—*lavender*, myrrh, patchouli, rose

Spiritual Uses

Align with the Divine—*angelica*, cinnamon, *grapefruit*, jasmine, *lemon, mandarin*, patchouli, rose, *sandalwood*, spikenard, thyme, ylang-ylang

Angel communication and connection—chamomile, *grapefruit*, jasmine, lavender, *mandarin*, melissa, rose, sage, spikenard

Ascended Masters—*angelica, benzoin*, bergamot, ginger, *grapefruit*, hyacinth, neroli

Atlantis—*bergamot, black pepper*, ginger, *grapefruit*, jasmine, lavender, *mandarin*, neroli, *orange, petitgrain*, rose, spikenard, sweet marjoram, thyme

Dreams (goals)—birch, *cinnamon, clove*, niaouli

Dreams (lucid, prophetic, and sleeping)—angelica, blue cypress, *chamomile*, ginger, *lavender, mandarin*, melissa, myrrh, ravensara

Intuition/psychic—angelica, anise seed, bergamot, black pepper, cardamom, *chamomile*, elemi, *frankincense*, lavender, melissa, palo santo, ravensara, sandalwood, spikenard

Life purpose—basil, benzoin, *black pepper*, niaouli, palmarosa, peppermint, pine, spikenard, spruce, thyme

Meditation—allspice, angelica, *benzoin*, bergamot, *cedarwood*, celery seed, chamomile, clary sage, coriander, elemi, *eucalyptus*, *frankincense*, ginger, *grapefruit*, lavender, *lemongrass*, hyacinth, palmarosa, palo santo, peppermint, petitgrain, rose, rosemary, *sage*, *sandalwood*, tea tree, *vetiver*, ylang-ylang

Mediumship—lavender, *myrrh*, neroli, *rosemary*

Miracles—jasmine, *rose*, *rosewood*, sandalwood

Past-life recall—*basil*, cardamom, cedarwood, coriander, ginger, juniper, *peppermint*, pine, rosewood, sage, *spruce*, thyme

Prayer—benzoin, cedarwood, celery seed, clary sage, lemongrass, patchouli, *sandalwood*, *spruce*, vetiver

Protection—*allspice*, anise seed, basil, benzoin, *cedarwood*, *clove*, eucalyptus, geranium, hyssop, myrrh, palmarosa, palo santo, pine, rosemary, sage, *sweet marjoram*

Shamanism—birch, *blue cypress*, *cedarwood*, chamomile, *juniper berry*, *palo santo*, patchouli, ravensara, *sage*, *spruce*, vetiver

Visualization—chamomile, clary sage, eucalyptus, *vetiver*

Totems, Animal

This section provides essential oil suggestions listed by animal totem as a quick and easy way to look up a list of oils that could work to petition the help and energetic vibration of animals and petition their assistance as an ally.

Alligator—niaouli

Angelfish—palmarosa

Antelope—black pepper

Bat—angelica

Bear—blue cypress, ravensara

Beaver—birch

Bee—lemongrass, melissa

Beetle—cedarwood

Butterfly—anise seed, melissa, peppermint

Camel—myrrh

Cat (domestic)—chamomile

Cat (kitten)—lavender

Clam—oregano

Coyote—lime

Crab—celery seed

Crow—palo santo, ravensara

Dog—hyssop, myrrh, palo santo, sweet marjoram

Dog (puppy)—lavender, orange, rosemary

Dolphin—basil, coriander, black pepper, tea tree

Dove—jasmine, rose, sweet marjoram, wintergreen, ylang-ylang

Dragon—hyssop, mandarin

Dragonfly—cedarwood, grapefruit, rosewood, spikenard

Eagle—allspice, chamomile, elemi, helichrysum

Earthworm—vetiver

Elephant—basil, cinnamon, frankincense, rosemary, sandalwood, spruce, thyme

Elk—spruce

Fish—spikenard

Fox—black pepper, grapefruit, lemon, lime, mandarin, peppermint, rosemary

Frog—coriander, niaouli

Goat—wintergreen

Goldfish—cinnamon

Gorilla—patchouli

Hawk—benzoin, cardamom, clove, helichrysum, melissa, niaouli, palmarosa, rosemary, rosewood, sandalwood, tea tree, thyme

Horse—clary sage, sweet marjoram

Hummingbird—bergamot, clary sage, ginger, lemon, lemongrass, lime, mandarin

Jellyfish—palmarosa

Koala—eucalyptus, hyacinth

Lion—orange, rosewood

Lizard—blue cypress, chamomile, mandarin, palo santo

Macaw Parrot (blue-and-gold)—lemon

Moth—anise seed

Mouse—sandalwood

Owl—benzoin, cinnamon, helichrysum, oregano, ravensara, rosemary

Parakeet—lemon

Peacock—birch, juniper berry, neroli, patchouli

Pelican—petitgrain

Phoenix—juniper berry

Porcupine—eucalyptus, fennel, pine

Rabbit—jasmine, wintergreen

Raven—benzoin, cinnamon, hyacinth, ravensara

Sloth—anise seed, basil, celery seed, fennel, grapefruit, lemon, melissa, peppermint

Snake—benzoin, celery seed, elemi, geranium, sage

Spider—bergamot, fennel, hyssop, palmarosa

Swan—rose

Turkey—allspice

Turtle—clove, pine, sage

Unicorn—angelica, rose, helichrysum

Vulture—cardamom

White Buffalo—basil, cedarwood, neroli, sandalwood, spruce

White Whale—basil, peppermint, thyme

Glossary of Therapeutic Qualities and Associated Oils

Abortifacient. Causes abortion. Basil, celery seed, clove, coriander, frankincense, hyssop, juniper berry, palmarosa, sage, vetiver.

Abrasions, protects and reduces bleeding. See astringent. Allspice, benzoin, birch, cedarwood, cinnamon, clary sage, eucalyptus, fennel, frankincense, geranium, ginger, grapefruit, hyssop, juniper berry, lemon, lemongrass, lime, mandarin, myrrh, neroli, orange, palmarosa, patchouli, peppermint, petitgrain, rose, rosemary, sage, sandalwood, spruce, thyme, vetiver, wintergreen.

Allergies, reduces. See antiallergenic. Eucalyptus, lavender, niaouli, ravensara.

Alterative. Restores healthy bodily functions. Patchouli, peppermint.

Analgesic. Relieves or reduces pain. Allspice, angelica, anise seed, basil, bergamot, birch, black pepper, celery seed, chamomile, cinnamon, clary sage, clove, coriander, blue cypress, elemi, eucalyptus, frankincense, geranium, ginger, helichrysum, jasmine, juniper berry, lavender, lemongrass, melissa, myrrh, neroli, niaouli, oregano, palmarosa, palo santo, patchouli, peppermint, pine, ravensara, rosemary, rosewood, sandalwood, spikenard, sweet marjoram, tea tree, thyme, vetiver, wintergreen.

Anaphrodisiac, Antaphrodisiac, or Anti-aphrodisiac. Reduces sexual desire. Oregano, sweet marjoram.

Anemia. See antianemic. Chamomile, lemon.

Anesthetic. Induces insensitivity to pain. Allspice, benzoin, birch, cinnamon, clove, coriander, peppermint, wintergreen.

Anthelmintic or Anthelminthic. Destroys and expels parasitic worms. Juniper berry, lavender, lemon, melissa, niaouli, oregano, palmarosa, peppermint, pine, sage, spikenard, thyme, vetiver.

Antiallergenic. Relieves or reduce allergy symptoms. Eucalyptus, lavender, niaouli, ravensara.

Antianemic. Prevents or readjusts anemia. Chamomile, lemon.

Antiarthritic. Relieves arthritic pain. Celery seed, blue cypress.

Antibacterial. Kills and inhibits the growth of bacteria; bactericidal. Angelica, basil, benzoin, black pepper, blue cypress, chamomile, cinnamon, clove, coriander, elemi, eucalyptus, fennel, frankincense, geranium, ginger, grapefruit, helichrysum, hyssop, jasmine, lavender, lemon, lemongrass, lime, melissa, neroli, orange, oregano, palmarosa, patchouli, peppermint, pine, ravensara, rosemary, rosewood, sage, sandalwood, spikenard, sweet marjoram, tea tree, thyme, vetiver, wintergreen.

Antibiotic. Prevents or kills bacterial growth. Basil, bergamot, chamomile, cinnamon, clove, eucalyptus, frankincense, geranium, lavender, lemon, melissa, oregano, patchouli, peppermint, ravensara, spikenard, tea tree, thyme.

Anticholinergic. Inhibits acetylcholine, a neurohormone of the parasympathetic nervous system responsible for everyday activities. Black pepper.

Anticoagulant. Retards or inhibits the coagulation of the blood. Birch, cinnamon, clove, fennel, geranium, ginger, helichrysum, orange, wintergreen.

Anticonvulsive. Relieves or prevents convulsions or epileptic seizures. Black pepper, celery seed, chamomile, cinnamon, clary sage, lavender, melissa, peppermint, rosewood, spikenard.

Antidepressant. Lessens, relieves, and prevents depression. Allspice, basil, benzoin, bergamot, chamomile, cinnamon, clary sage, clove, frankincense, geranium, grapefruit, helichrysum, hyacinth, jasmine, lavender, lemon, lemongrass, lime, mandarin, melissa, neroli, orange, patchouli, peppermint, petitgrain, rosemary, rosewood, sage, sandalwood, thyme, ylang-ylang.

Antidiabetic. Lowers glucose levels. Cinnamon, eucalyptus, geranium, myrrh, sage.

Antidiarrheal. Stops or provides relief from diarrhea. Cinnamon, peppermint.

Antidote. Counteracts a poison. Black pepper, cinnamon, eucalyptus, fennel, ginger.

Antiemetic. Reduces and discontinues nausea and vomiting. Anise seed, black pepper, chamomile, cinnamon, clove, fennel, ginger, mandarin, orange, oregano, patchouli.

Antifungal. Destroys fungus; fungicide. Angelica, chamomile, cinnamon, clove, elemi, eucalyptus, fennel, geranium, helichrysum, jasmine, juniper berry, lavender, lemon, lemongrass, myrrh, neroli, orange, oregano, palmarosa, patchouli, pine, rosemary, rosewood, sage, sandalwood, spikenard, sweet marjoram, tea tree, thyme.

Antigalactagogue. Reduces milk production; suppresses lactation. Peppermint, sage.

Anti-infectious. Prevents and reduces infections. Ravensara, sandalwood, tea tree.

Anti-inflammatory. Diminishes and calms inflammation. Angelica, benzoin, birch, blue cypress, cardamom, chamomile, cinnamon, clary sage, clove, coriander, eucalyptus, frankincense, geranium, ginger, helichrysum, hyssop, jasmine, juniper berry, lavender, melissa, myrrh, orange, oregano, palo santo, patchouli, sage, sandalwood, spikenard, spruce, tea tree, thyme, vetiver, wintergreen.

Antilithic. Prevents the formation of kidney stones or promotes their dissolution. Celery seed, juniper berry, lemon, lime.

Antimicrobial. Destroys or inhibits the growth of disease-causing microorganisms. Cardamom, lemongrass, palo santo, tea tree, thyme.

Antimutagenic. Reduces the frequency of mutation or interferes with the mutagenic effects of another substance. Benzoin, coriander.

Antineuralgic. Relieves or stops nerve pain. Chamomile, clove, eucalyptus, geranium, lemon, peppermint, pine, rosemary.

Antioxidant. Inhibits oxidation and counteracts deterioration of living organisms. Allspice, benzoin, celery seed, cinnamon, clove, coriander, frankincense, ginger, lemon, lime, melissa, rosemary, sage, spikenard, sweet marjoram, thyme.

Antiparasitic. Used for treatment of parasitic diseases like nematodes and infectious protozoa. Basil, benzoin, bergamot, birch, cardamom, chamomile, cinnamon, clove, eucalyptus, fennel, geranium, ginger, hyssop, juniper berry, lavender, lemon, melissa, niaouli, oregano, palmarosa, patchouli, peppermint, pine, rosemary, rosewood, sage, spikenard, spruce, tea tree, thyme, vetiver.

Antiperspirant. Prevents or reduces perspiration. Lemongrass.

Antiphlogistic. Counteracts inflammation. Celery seed, fennel, patchouli, peppermint, pine, sandalwood.

Antipruritic. Relieves and inhibits itching. Benzoin, cedarwood, chamomile, eucalyptus, jasmine, lemon, peppermint, sandalwood, tea tree, thyme, ylang-ylang.

Antiputrid. Stops and slows down decay or rotting of the body or other organic matter. Cinnamon, eucalyptus, melissa, myrrh, thyme.

Antipyorrhea. Reduces the infection and inflammation of gums or periodontitis. Myrrh, orange.

Antipyretic. Reduces fever. See febrifugal.

Antirheumatic. Reduces and slows the progression of rheumatoid arthritis. Angelica, birch, celery seed, chamomile, cinnamon, clove, coriander, eucalyptus, hyssop, juniper berry, lavender, lemon, lime, niaouli, oregano, pine, rosemary, sage, thyme, wintergreen.

Antisclerotic. Prevents hardening of tissue. Lemon, lime.

Antiscorbutic. Prevents or cures scurvy, a vitamin C deficiency. Celery seed, ginger, juniper berry, lemon, lime, orange, pine.

Antiseborrheic. Reduces or prevents excessive sebum production. Cedarwood.

Antiseptic. Prevents and kills the growth of disease-causing microorganisms. Allspice, angelica, anise seed, basil, benzoin, bergamot, birch, black pepper, cardamom, cedarwood, chamomile, cinnamon, clary sage, clove, elemi, eucalyptus, fennel, frankincense, geranium, ginger, grapefruit, helichrysum, hyacinth, hyssop, jasmine, juniper berry, lavender, lemon, lemongrass, lime, mandarin, melissa, myrrh, neroli, niaouli, orange, oregano, palmarosa, patchouli, peppermint, petitgrain, pine, ravensara, rosemary, rosewood, sage, sandalwood, spikenard, spruce, sweet marjoram, tea tree, thyme, vetiver, wintergreen, ylang-ylang.

Antispasmodic. Alleviates and prevents spasms, cramps, and convulsions. Angelica, anise seed, basil, benzoin, bergamot, black pepper, cardamom, cedarwood, celery seed, chamomile, cinnamon, clary sage, clove, coriander, eucalyptus, fennel, frankincense, geranium, ginger, helichrysum, hyssop, jasmine, juniper berry, lavender, lemon, lime, mandarin, melissa, myrrh, neroli, niaouli, orange, oregano, palmarosa, petitgrain, pine, ravensara, rosemary, sage, sandalwood, spikenard, spruce, sweet marjoram, thyme, vetiver, wintergreen.

Antistress. Reduces stress. Basil, benzoin, bergamot, clary sage, clove, geranium, grapefruit, jasmine, lavender, lemon, mandarin, melissa, neroli, orange, palmarosa, patchouli, petitgrain, sandalwood, sweet marjoram, vetiver.

Antisudorific. Stops or prevents sweating. Clary sage, sage.

Antitoxic. Neutralizes and counteracts poisons. Bergamot, birch, black pepper, chamomile, fennel, ginger, grapefruit, juniper berry, lavender, lemon, lime, orange, oregano, patchouli, peppermint, ravensara, rosemary, thyme.

Antitumor. Prevents the formation or growth of tumors. Coriander.

Antitussive. Prevents and gets rid of coughs. Angelica, anise seed, basil, benzoin, bergamot, black pepper, cardamom, cedarwood, cinnamon, clove, elemi, eucalyptus, fennel, frankincense, ginger, helichrysum, hyssop, jasmine, juniper berry, lavender, lemon, mandarin, myrrh, niaouli, orange, oregano, peppermint, pine, ravensara, rosemary, sage, sandalwood, spruce, sweet marjoram, tea tree, thyme, wintergreen.

Antivenomous. An antidote to poisons and bites from insects and snakes. Basil, eucalyptus, lavender, thyme.

Antiviral. Removes, kills, and protects against viruses. Angelica, benzoin, blue cypress, cinnamon, clary sage, clove, elemi, eucalyptus, grapefruit, helichrysum, hyssop, jasmine, lavender, lemon, lemongrass, lime, melissa, neroli, orange, oregano, palmarosa, patchouli, peppermint, petitgrain, pine, ravensara, rosemary, rosewood, sage, sandalwood, sweet marjoram, tea tree, thyme.

Anxiety, reduces. See sedative. Anise seed, bergamot, chamomile, clary sage, fennel, jasmine, lavender, lemon, mandarin, melissa, neroli, orange, palmarosa, patchouli, petitgrain, rosewood, sandalwood, spikenard, sweet marjoram, vetiver.

Aperitive. Stimulates the appetite. Angelica, anise seed, basil, bergamot, black pepper, celery seed, chamomile, cinnamon, clove, coriander, fennel, ginger, grapefruit, lavender, lemon, lime, mandarin, melissa, myrrh, orange, oregano, palmarosa, peppermint, sage, spikenard, thyme.

Aphrodisiac. Stimulates sexual desire. Allspice, angelica, basil, benzoin, black pepper, cardamom, celery seed, cinnamon, clary sage, clove, coriander, ginger, hyacinth, jasmine, juniper berry, neroli, palmarosa, patchouli, peppermint, rosemary, rosewood, sandalwood, thyme, vetiver, ylang-ylang.

Appetite, increases. See aperitive and stomachic. Allspice, angelica, anise seed, basil, bergamot, black pepper, cardamom, celery seed, chamomile, cinnamon, clary sage, clove, coriander, elemi, fennel, ginger, hyssop, juniper berry, lavender, lemon, mandarin, melissa, myrrh, orange, oregano, patchouli, peppermint, petitgrain, rosemary, sage, sandalwood, sweet marjoram, thyme, vetiver.

Astringent. Contracts body tissues to protect the skin and to reduce bleeding from minor abrasions. Allspice, benzoin, birch, cedarwood, cinnamon, clary sage, eucalyptus, fennel, frankincense, geranium, ginger, grapefruit, helichrysum, hyssop, juniper berry, lemon, lemongrass, lime, mandarin, myrrh, neroli, orange, palmarosa, patchouli, peppermint, petitgrain, rose, rosemary, sage, sandalwood, spruce, thyme, vetiver, wintergreen.

Bacteria, destroys or inhibits. See antibacterial and antibiotic. Angelica, basil, blue cypress, cinnamon, clove, coriander, elemi, eucalyptus, fennel, frankincense, geranium, ginger, grapefruit, hyssop, jasmine, lemon, melissa, oregano, geranium, patchouli, peppermint, ravensara, spikenard, tea tree, thyme.

Balancing. Stablize, harmonize, and promote health. Ginger, grapefruit.

Balsamic. Softens and reduces mucus. Cedarwood, cinnamon, clary sage, coriander, elemi, frankincense, hyssop, oregano, spikenard, thyme.

Bile, produces and discharges. See cholagogic. Celery seed, chamomile, grapefruit, juniper berry, lavender, mandarin, orange, oregano, peppermint, pine, ravensara, rose, rosemary, sage.

Bile, secretion. See choleretic. Melissa, orange, oregano, pine, ravensara, rosemary.

Bleeding, stops. See hemostatic. Cinnamon, eucalyptus, geranium, grapefruit, juniper berry, lemon, lime, myrrh, orange, sage, spruce, wintergreen.

Blood pressure, decreases. See vasodilator and hypotensor. Black pepper, rose, sweet marjoram.

Blood pressure, increases. See vasoconstrictor and hyperstensor. Geranium, orange, peppermint.

Blood purifier. See depurative. Angelica, basil, birch, celery seed, coriander, eucalyptus, fennel, geranium, grapefruit, hyssop, juniper berry, lemon, lime, mandarin, myrrh, neroli, orange, peppermint, pine, sage, spikenard.

Blood sugar, lowers. See hypoglycemient. Anise seed, cinnamon, myrrh.

Calmative. Elicits a sedative effect. Anise seed, bergamot, chamomile, clary sage, coriander, fennel, jasmine, lavender, lemon, mandarin, melissa, neroli, orange, palmarosa, patchouli, petitgrain, rosewood, sandalwood, spikenard, sweet marjoram, vetiver, ylang-ylang.

Calms nerves. See nervine. Angelica, basil, celery seed, chamomile, clary sage, coriander, elemi, frankincense, hyssop, juniper berry, lavender, lemongrass, melissa, orange, palmarosa, patchouli, peppermint, petitgrain, rosemary, sage, spikenard, sweet marjoram, thyme, vetiver, ylang-ylang.

Cardiac. Affects the heart. Anise seed, black pepper, cinnamon, hyssop, thyme.

Cardiotonic. Stimulates and tones the heart. Coriander, spikenard, vetiver.

Carminative. Relieves and expels excess gas. Allspice, angelica, anise seed, basil, benzoin, bergamot, black pepper, cardamom, celery seed, chamomile, cinnamon, clary sage, clove, coriander, fennel, frankincense, ginger, hyssop, jasmine, juniper berry, lavender, lemon, lemongrass, mandarin, melissa, myrrh, neroli, orange, oregano, palmarosa, patchouli, peppermint, ravensara, rosemary, sage, sandalwood, spikenard, sweet marjoram, tea tree, thyme, vetiver, wintergreen, ylang-ylang.

Caustic. Corrodes organic tissue by chemical action. Clove.

Cephalic. Of, in, or relating to the head. Angelica, basil, benzoin, cardamom, eucalyptus, frankincense, ginger, grapefruit, helichrysum, hyssop, lavender, lemon, melissa, peppermint, rosemary, rosewood, sweet marjoram.

Childbirth, facilitates. See parturient. Clary sage, fennel, geranium, helichrysum, jasmine, sage, ylang-ylang.

Cholagogic. Promotes the production and discharge of bile. Celery seed, chamomile, grapefruit, helichrysum, juniper berry, lavender, mandarin, orange, oregano, peppermint, pine, ravensara, rose, rosemary, sage.

Choleretic. Stimulates the liver to promote bile secretion. Melissa, orange, oregano, pine, ravensara, rosemary.

Cicatrizant. Helps the formation of scar tissue. Angelica, benzoin, bergamot, chamomile, clove, elemi, eucalyptus, frankincense, geranium, helichrysum, hyssop, jasmine, juniper berry, lavender, lemon, myrrh, neroli, niaouli, palmarosa, patchouli, rosemary, sage, sandalwood, tea tree, thyme.

Coagulant. Changes the blood to a solid or semi-solid state. Lemon.

Congestion, reduces. See decongestant. Eucalyptus, fennel, jasmine, lavender, lemon, mandarin, niaouli, patchouli, peppermint, pine, rosemary, sandalwood, sweet marjoram, tea tree, wintergreen.

Constipation, relieves. See laxative and purgative. Basil, benzoin, bergamot, birch, black pepper, chamomile, fennel, frankincense, ginger, hyssop, lemon, orange, oregano, patchouli, pine, rosemary, sage, spikenard, sweet marjoram.

Convulsions, relieves. See anticonvulsive. Black pepper, celery seed, chamomile, cinnamon, clary sage, lavender, melissa, peppermint, rosewood, spikenard.

Cooling. Relieves over-exertion, reduces heat and over-excitement. Eucalyptus, lemon, lime, myrrh.

Cordial. Revives, stimulates, and invigorates. Benzoin, bergamot, lavender, neroli, peppermint, sweet marjoram, tea tree.

Coughs, relieves. See antitussive. Angelica, anise seed, basil, benzoin, bergamot, black pepper, cardamom, cedarwood, cinnamon, clove, elemi, eucalyptus, fennel, frankincense, ginger, helichrysum, hyssop, jasmine, juniper berry, lavender, lemon, mandarin, myrrh, niaouli, orange, oregano, peppermint, pine, ravensara, rosemary, sage, sandalwood, spruce, sweet marjoram, tea tree, thyme, wintergreen.

Counter-irritant. Creates inflammation in one location with the goal of lessening the inflammation in another location. Thyme.

Cytophylactic. Prevents the disintegration of a cell by rupture and protects the cell wall or membrane. Frankincense, geranium, helichrysum, lavender, mandarin, melissa, neroli, oregano, palmarosa, patchouli, rosemary, thyme.

Decay, reduces and slows. See antiputrid. Cinnamon, eucalyptus, melissa, myrrh, thyme.

Decongestant. Relieves congestion in the upper respiratory tract. Eucalyptus, fennel, jasmine, lavender, lemon, mandarin, niaouli, patchouli, peppermint, pine, rosemary, sandalwood, sweet marjoram, tea tree, wintergreen.

Deodorizer. Removes or conceals unpleasant smells. Benzoin, bergamot, clary sage, coriander, eucalyptus, geranium, lavender, lemongrass, myrrh, neroli, patchouli, petitgrain, pine, rosewood, sandalwood, spikenard.

Depression, relieves. See antidepressant. Allspice, basil, benzoin, bergamot, chamomile, cinnamon, clary sage, clove, frankincense, geranium, grapefruit, helichrysum, hyacinth, jasmine, lavender, lemon, lemongrass, lime, mandarin, melissa, neroli, orange, patchouli, peppermint, petitgrain, rosemary, rosewood, sage, sandalwood, thyme, ylang-ylang.

Depurative. Purifies the blood and internal organs. Angelica, birch, celery seed, coriander, eucalyptus, fennel, geranium, grapefruit, hyssop, juniper berry, lemon, lime, mandarin, myrrh, orange, peppermint, pine, sage, spikenard.

Dermatological. Healing and maintenance for the skin. Clove (anti-inflammatory).

Detersive. Cleanses; a detergent. Birch.

Detoxifier. Removes or reduces toxins from the body. Black pepper, coriander, fennel, grapefruit, helichrysum, juniper berry, lavender, lemon, peppermint, rosemary, sweet marjoram, vetiver.

Diabetes, lowers glucose. See antidiabetic. Cinnamon, eucalyptus, geranium, myrrh, sage.

Diaphoretic. Increases and induces perspiration. Angelica, basil, black pepper, celery seed, chamomile, coriander, eucalyptus, fennel, ginger, hyssop, lemon, melissa, niaouli, oregano, patchouli, rosemary, sandalwood, spruce, sweet marjoram, tea tree, thyme, vetiver.

Digestion, promotes. See digestive. Allspice, angelica, anise seed, basil, bergamot, black pepper, cardamom, celery seed, chamomile, cinnamon, clary sage, coriander, fennel, frankincense, ginger, grapefruit, hyssop, juniper berry, lemon, lime, mandarin, melissa, neroli, orange, palmarosa, patchouli, peppermint, petitgrain, rose, rosemary, sage, spikenard, sweet marjoram, thyme.

Digestive. Stimulates the secretion of digestive juices; promotes and aids digestion. Allspice, angelica, anise seed, basil, bergamot, black pepper, cardamom, celery seed, chamomile, cinnamon, clary sage, coriander, fennel, frankincense, ginger, grapefruit, hyssop, juniper berry, lemon, lime, mandarin, melissa, neroli, orange, palmarosa, patchouli, peppermint, petitgrain, rose, rosemary, sage, spikenard, sweet marjoram, thyme.

Disinfectant. Destroys bacteria. Benzoin, birch, eucalyptus, lemon, lime, niaouli, oregano, rosemary, sage, tea tree.

Diuretic. Increases excretion of urine. Angelica, anise seed, benzoin, birch, black pepper, cardamom, cedarwood, celery seed, chamomile, coriander, eucalyptus, fennel, frankincense, geranium, ginger, grapefruit, helichrysum, hyssop, juniper berry, lavender, lemon, lemongrass, mandarin, myrrh, orange, oregano, palo santo, patchouli, pine, ravensara, rose, rosemary, sage, sandalwood, spikenard, spruce, sweet marjoram, thyme, vetiver, wintergreen.

Drying. Hardening through exposure to air. Benzoin, myrrh.

Emetic. Induces vomiting. Vetiver.

Emmenagogic. Stimulates or increases menstrual flow and encourages expulsion of the uterine contents. Angelica, anise seed, basil, cedarwood, celery seed, chamomile, cinnamon, clary sage, clove, coriander, fennel, frankincense, ginger, hyssop, jasmine, juniper berry, lavender, melissa, myrrh, oregano, palmarosa, peppermint, rosemary, sage, spikenard, sweet marjoram, thyme, vetiver, wintergreen, ylang-ylang.

Emollient. Softens or smooths the skin. Cedarwood, chamomile, cinnamon, clary sage, frankincense, hyssop, jasmine, lemon, mandarin, neroli, palmarosa, rosewood, sandalwood, ylang-ylang.

Estrogenic. Having properties similar to estrogen; estrus-producing. Angelica, basil, cinnamon, clary sage, fennel, sage.

Euphoriant. Produces a feeling of euphoria. Benzoin, clary sage, jasmine, neroli, rosewood, sage, sandalwood, spruce, ylang-ylang.

Expectorant. See antitussive. Angelica, anise seed, basil, benzoin, bergamot, black pepper, cardamom, cedarwood, cinnamon, clove, elemi, eucalyptus, fennel, frankincense, ginger, helichrysum, hyssop, jasmine, juniper berry, lavender, lemon, mandarin, myrrh, niaouli, orange, oregano, peppermint, pine, ravensara, rosemary, sage, sandalwood, spruce, sweet marjoram, tea tree, thyme, wintergreen.

Febrifugal. Reduces fevers. Angelica, basil, bergamot, birch, black pepper, cinnamon, coriander, eucalyptus, ginger, hyssop, lemon, lemongrass, lime, melissa, niaouli, orange, oregano, palmarosa, patchouli, peppermint, ravensara, sage, sandalwood, spikenard, sweet marjoram, thyme.

Fever, reduces. See febrifugal. Angelica, basil, bergamot, birch, black pepper, cinnamon, coriander, eucalyptus, ginger, hyssop, lemon, lemongrass, lime, melissa, niaouli, orange, oregano, palmarosa, patchouli, peppermint, ravensara, sage, sandalwood, spikenard, sweet marjoram, thyme.

Fixative. Stabilizes volatility and preserves a synergistic blend. Benzoin, blue cypress, clary sage, elemi, frankincense, myrrh, patchouli, petitgrain, sandalwood, spikenard, vetiver, ylang-ylang.

Fungus, destroys. See antifungal. Angelica, chamomile, cinnamon, clove, elemi, eucalyptus, fennel, geranium, helichrysum, jasmine, juniper berry, lavender, lemon, lemongrass, myrrh, neroli, orange, oregano, palmarosa, patchouli, pine, rosemary, rosewood, sage, sandalwood, spikenard, sweet marjoram, tea tree, thyme.

Galactagogic. Induces milk secretion. Anise seed, basil, fennel, jasmine, lemongrass, melissa, sweet marjoram, wintergreen.

Gas or flatulence, reduces and expels. See carminative. Allspice, angelica, anise seed, basil, benzoin, bergamot, black pepper, cardamom, celery seed, chamomile, cinnamon, clary sage, clove, coriander, fennel, frankincense, ginger, hyssop, jasmine, juniper berry, lavender, lemon, lemongrass, mandarin, melissa, myrrh, neroli, orange, oregano, palmarosa, patchouli, peppermint, ravensara, rosemary, sage, sandalwood, spikenard, sweet marjoram, tea tree, thyme, vetiver, wintergreen, ylang-ylang.

Germicide. Destroys harmful microrganisms; antiseptic, antimicrobial, disinfectant. Eucalyptus, jasmine, juniper berry.

Gums, inflammation. See antipyorrhea. Myrrh, orange.

Healing. The process of making or becoming healthy again. Cedarwood, clary sage, geranium, lavender, and essentially all oils.

Hemostatic. Stops bleeding. Cinnamon, eucalyptus, geranium, grapefruit, juniper berry, lemon, lime, myrrh, orange, sage, spruce, wintergreen.

Hepatic. Affects or drains the liver. Angelica, celery seed, chamomile, cinnamon, coriander, fennel, helichrysum, lemon, lime, orange, oregano, peppermint, rose, rosemary, sage, spikenard.

Hypertensor. Raises blood pressure. Hyssop, pine, rosemary, sage, thyme.

Hypnotic. Induces sleep. Hyacinth, mandarin, neroli, orange, oregano.

Hypoglycemient. Lowers blood-sugar levels. Anise seed, cinnamon, myrrh.

Hypotensor. Lowers blood pressure. Celery seed, chamomile, clary sage, lavender, lemon, melissa, neroli, sweet marjoram, wintergreen, ylang-ylang.

Infections, prevents and reduces. See anti-infectious. Ravensara, sandalwood, tea tree.

Inflammation, reduces. See antiphlogistic. Celery seed, fennel, patchouli, peppermint, pine, sandalwood.

Insect bites, poisonous antidote. See antivenomous. Basil, eucalyptus, lavender, thyme.

Insecticidal. Destroys or controls insects. Basil, benzoin, bergamot, birch, black pepper, blue cypress, cedarwood, cinnamon, clove, eucalyptus, fennel, geranium, juniper berry, lavender, lemon, lemongrass, lime, melissa, niaouli, palo santo, peppermint, patchouli, pine, rosemary, rosewood, sage, sandalwood, tea tree, thyme, vetiver.

Insects, controls or destroys. See insecticidal. Basil, benzoin, bergamot, birch, black pepper, blue cypress, cedarwood, cinnamon, clove, eucalyptus, fennel, geranium, juniper berry, lavender, lemon, lemongrass, lime, melissa, niaouli, palo santo, peppermint, patchouli, pine, rosemary, rosewood, sage, sandalwood, tea tree, thyme, vetiver.

Invigorating. Increases energy, strength, and good health. Eucaplytus, lemon, myrrh, peppermint, rosemary, spruce.

Itching, relieves. See antipruritic. Benzoin, cedarwood, chamomile, eucalyptus, jasmine, lemon, peppermint, sandalwood, tea tree, thyme, ylang-ylang.

Kidney stones, prevents and dissolves. See antilithic. Celery seed, juniper berry, lemon, lime.

Laxative. Stimulates the evacuation of the bowels. Basil, benzoin, bergamot, birch, black pepper, chamomile, fennel, ginger, hyssop, lemon, orange, oregano, patchouli, pine, rosemary, sage, spikenard, sweet marjoram.

Liver, drains. See hepatic. Angelica, celery seed, chamomile, cinnamon, coriander, fennel, helichrysum, lemon, lime, orange, oregano, peppermint, rose, rosemary, sage, spikenard.

Menstrual flow, increases. See emmenagogic. Angelica, anise seed, basil, cedarwood, celery seed, chamomile, cinnamon, clary sage, clove, coriander, fennel, frankincense, ginger, hyssop, jasmine, juniper berry, lavender, melissa, myrrh, oregano, palmarosa, peppermint, rosemary, sage, spikenard, sweet marjoram, thyme, vetiver, wintergreen, ylang-ylang.

Milk secretion. See galactagogic. Anise seed, basil, fennel, jasmine, lemongrass, melissa, sweet marjoram, wintergreen.

Moisturizer. Ylang-ylang.

Mucus, reduces. See balsamic. Cedarwood, cinnamon, clary sage, coriander, elemi, frankincense, hyssop, oregano, spikenard, thyme.

Narcotic. Relieves pain and soothes; induces sleep. Clary sage.

Nausea, reduces. See antiemetic. Black pepper, chamomile, cinnamon, clove, fennel, ginger, mandarin, orange, patchouli.

Nerve pain, reduces. See antineuralgic. Chamomile, clove, eucalyptus, geranium, lemon, peppermint, pine, rosemary.

Nervine. Calms the nerves. Angelica, basil, celery seed, chamomile, clary sage, coriander, elemi, frankincense, helichrysum, hyssop, juniper berry, lavender, lemongrass, melissa, orange, palmarosa, patchouli, peppermint, petitgrain, rosemary, sage, spikenard, spruce, sweet marjoram, thyme, vetiver, ylang-ylang.

Oily skin, reduces. See antiseborrheic. Cedarwood.

Pain, reduces. See analgesic. Allspice, angelica, anise seed, basil, bergamot, birch, black pepper, celery seed, chamomile, cinnamon, clary sage, clove, coriander, blue cypress, elemi, eucalyptus, frankincense, geranium, ginger, helichrysum, jasmine, juniper berry, lavender, lemongrass, melissa, myrrh, neroli, niaouli, oregano, palmarosa, palo santo, patchouli, peppermint, pine, ravensara, rosemary, rosewood, sandalwood, spikenard, sweet marjoram, tea tree, thyme, vetiver, wintergreen.

Parasites, reduces. See antiparasitic. Basil, benzoin, bergamot, birch, cardamom, chamomile, cinnamon, clove, eucalyptus, fennel, geranium, ginger, hyssop, juniper berry, lavender, lemon, melissa, niaouli, oregano, palmarosa, patchouli, peppermint, pine, rosemary, rosewood, sage, spikenard, spruce, tea tree, thyme, vetiver.

Parturient. Facilitates labor and childbirth. Clary sage, fennel, geranium, jasmine, sage, ylang-ylang.

Perspiration, increases. See diaphorectic and sudorific. Angelica, basil, chamomile, hyssop, juniper berry, lavender, myrrh, oregano, palmarosa, peppermint, pine, rosemary, tea tree, thyme.

Poison, neutralizes and counteracts. See antitoxic. Bergamot, birch, black pepper, chamomile, fennel, ginger, grapefruit, juniper berry, lavender, lemon, lime, orange, oregano, patchouli, peppermint, ravensara, rosemary, thyme.

Preservative. Counteracts decaying, decomposition, or fermentation. Benzoin, cinnamon, euacalyptus, melissa, myrrh, thyme.

Purgative. A laxative; evacuant. Frankincense.

Purifying. Cleanses and decontaminates. Eucalyptus, grapefruit, lemon.

Refreshing. Invigorate or reinvigorate to make fresh, new, or different. Bergamot, clary sage, coriander, juniper berry, lemon, lime, orange, palmarosa, petitgrain, pine, tea tree.

Regenerative (skin). Benzoin, cedarwood, clary sage, eucalyptus, frankincense, geranium, grapefruit, helochrysum, jasmine, lavender, lemongrass, myrrh, neroli, niaouli, palmarosa, patchouli, rose, rosemary, rosewood, ylang-ylang.

Regenerator. Promotes new growth. Restores and repairs structure or tissue. Coriander, helichrysum.

Rejuvenator. Restores youthfulness. Benzoin, frankincense, geranium, helichrysum, myrrh, ylang-ylang.

Relaxant. Promotes relief of stress and tension; relaxes. Allspice, clary sage, myrrh, neroli, sandalwood, spikenard, ylang-ylang.

Resolvent. Reduces inflammation or swelling. Fennel, grapefruit, hyssop.

Restorative. Renews health and strength. Basil, geranium, grapefruit, lavender, lime, palo santo, peppermint, pine, sweet marjoram.

Revitalizing. Encourages vitality; re-energizes and regenerates. Angelica, coriander, fennel, frankincense, mandarin, myrrh (skin), tea tree, vetiver.

Reviving. Restores strength and energy; revitalizes. Grapefruit, lavender, niaouli, pine.

Rheumatoid arthritis, reduces. See antirheumatic. Angelica, birch, celery seed, chamomile, cinnamon, clove, coriander, eucalyptus, hyssop, juniper berry, lavender, lemon, lime, niaouli, oregano, pine, rosemary, sage, thyme, wintergreen.

Rubefacient. An irritant that reddens the skin. Allspice, bergamot, birch, black pepper, eucalyptus, ginger, juniper berry, lemon, oregano, pine, rosemary, spruce, thyme, vetiver, wintergreen.

Scar, promotes formation. See cicatrizant. Angelica, benzoin, bergamot, chamomile, clove, elemi, eucalyptus, frankincense, geranium, helichrysum, hyssop, jasmine, juniper berry, lavender, lemon, myrrh, neroli, niaouli, palmarosa, patchouli, rosemary, sage, sandalwood, tea tree, thyme.

Sedative. Promotes calm, reduces anxiety, and induces sleep. Allspice, anise seed, basil, benzoin, bergamot, black pepper, blue cypress, cedarwood, celery seed, chamomile, clary sage, fennel, frankincense, geranium, helichrysum, hyacinth, jasmine, juniper berry, lavender, lemon, lemongrass, mandarin, melissa, myrrh, neroli, orange, palmarosa, patchouli, petitgrain, ravensara, rosewood, sandalwood, spikenard, spruce, sweet marjoram, thyme, vetiver, ylang-ylang.

Sexual desire, increases. See aphrodisiac. Black pepper, ginger, hyacinth, jasmine, juniper berry, neroli, palmarosa, patchouli, peppermint, rosemary, rosewood, sandalwood, thyme, vetiver, ylang-ylang.

Sexual desire, reduces. See anaphrodisiac. Oregano, sweet marjoram.

Sleep, induces. See narcotic and sedative. Anise seed, bergamot, chamomile, clary sage, fennel, jasmine, lavender, lemon, mandarin, melissa, neroli, orange, palmarosa, patchouli, petitgrain, rosewood, sandalwood, spikenard, sweet marjoram, vetiver.

Snake bites, antidote. See antivenomous.

Soothing. Encourages calmness. Benzoin, lavender.

Spasms, alleviates. See antispasmodic. Angelica, anise seed, basil, benzoin, bergamot, cardamom, cedarwood, celery seed, chamomile, cinnamon, clary sage, clove, coriander, eucalyptus, fennel, frankincense, geranium, ginger, helichrysum, hyssop, jasmine, juniper berry, lavender, lemon, lime, mandarin, melissa, myrrh, neroli, niaouli, orange, sandalwood, spikenard, spruce, sweet marjoram, thyme, vetiver, wintergreen.

Stimulative. A restorative to raise levels of activity in the body. Allspice, angelica, anise seed, basil, benzoin, birch, black pepper, cardamom, celery seed, cinnamon, clary sage, clove, coriander, elemi, eucalyptus, fennel, frankincense, geranium, ginger, grapefruit, hyssop, jasmine, juniper berry, lavender, lemon, lime, mandarin, myrrh, niaouli, orange, oregano, palmarosa, patchouli, peppermint, petitgrain, pine, ravensara, rosemary, rosewood, sage, sandalwood, tea tree, thyme, vetiver, wintergreen, ylang-ylang.

Stomachic. Assists digestion; increases the appetite; tones the stomach. Allspice, angelica, anise seed, basil, bergamot, black pepper, cardamom, celery seed, chamomile, cinnamon, clary sage, clove, coriander, elemi, fennel, ginger, hyssop, juniper berry, lavender, lemon, mandarin, melissa, myrrh, orange, oregano, patchouli, peppermint, petitgrain, rosemary, sage, sandalwood, sweet marjoram, thyme, vetiver.

Sudorific. Induces sweating. Angelica, basil, chamomile, hyssop, juniper berry, lavender, myrrh, oregano, palmarosa, peppermint, pine, rosemary, tea tree, thyme.

Sweating. See perspiration. Angelica, benzoin, blue cypress, cinnamon, clove, elemi, eucalyptus, helichrysum, hyssop, jasmine, lavender, lime, melissa, orange, oregano, palmarosa, patchouli, peppermint, pine, ravensara, rosemary, rosewood, sage, sandalwood, sweet marjoram, tea tree, thyme.

Tonic. A stimulant restorative substance that increases vitality and well-being. Allspice, angelica, basil, benzoin, bergamot, birch, black pepper, cardamom, celery seed, chamomile, cinnamon, clary sage, clove, coriander, elemi, eucalyptus, fennel, helichrysum, neroli, niaouli, orange, oregano, palmarosa, patchouli, peppermint, petitgrain, pine, ravensara, rose, rosemary, rosewood, sage, sandalwood, spikenard, spruce, sweet marjoram, thyme, vetiver, wintergreen, ylang-ylang.

Tonifying. Increases energy to an organ or system of the body. Black pepper, clary sage, frankincense, geranium, ginger, grapefruit, juniper berry, myrrh.

Uplifting. Elevates moods; inspires; encourages happiness. Benzoin, bergamot, clary sage, clove, coriander, eucalyptus, frankincense, geranium, jasmine, lemon, lime, mandarin, melissa, neroli, palmarosa, patchouli, peppermint, petitgrain, rosemary, rosewood, thyme.

Vasoconstrictor. Constricts or narrows blood vessels, which increases blood pressure. Geranium, orange, peppermint.

Vasodilator. Dilates or widens blood vessels, which decreases blood pressure. Black pepper, rose, sweet marjoram.

Virus, removes and protects from. See antiviral. Angelica, benzoin, blue cypress, cinnamon, clove, elemi, eucalyptus, helichrysum, hyssop, jasmine, lavender, lime, melissa, orange, oregano, palmarosa, patchouli, peppermint, pine, ravensara, rosemary, rosewood, sage, sandalwood, sweet marjoram, tea tree, thyme.

Vitality, restores. See stimulative and tonic. Allspice, angelica, anise seed, basil, benzoin, birch, black pepper, cardamom, celery seed, cinnamon, clove, coriander, elemi, eucalyptus, fennel, frankincense, geranium, ginger, grapefruit, hyssop, jasmine, juniper berry, lavender, lemon, lime, myrrh, niaouli, orange, oregano, palmarosa, patchouli, peppermint, petitgrain, pine, ravensara, sage, sandalwood, tea tree, thyme, vetiver, wintergreen, ylang-ylang.

Vomiting, induces. See emetic. Vetiver.

Vomiting, lessens or prevents. See antiemetic. Black pepper, chamomile, cinnamon, clove, fennel, ginger, mandarin, orange, patchouli.

Vulnerary. Heals wounds. Benzoin, bergamot, celery seed, chamomile, elemi, eucalyptus, frankincense, geranium, hyssop, juniper berry, lavender, melissa, myrrh, niaouli, orange, oregano, pine, rosemary, sage, spruce, sweet marjoram, tea tree, wintergreen.

Warming. Clary sage, coriander, frankincense, oregano, rosemary, sage, sprice, sweet marjoram, thyme.

Wounds, heals. See vulnerary. Benzoin, bergamot, celery seed, chamomile, elemi, eucalyptus, frankincense, geranium, hyssop, juniper berry, lavender, melissa, myrrh, niaouli, orange, oregano, pine, rosemary, sage, spruce, sweet marjoram, tea tree, wintergreen.

Recommended Reading

Animal-Speak by Ted Andrews. Llewellyn Publications, 1993.

Animal-Wise by Ted Andrews. Dragonhawk, 1999.

Astrology by Isabel Hickey. Isabel Hickey, 1970.

Bach Flower Therapy Theory and Practice by Mechthild Scheffer. Healing Arts Press, 1988.

Chakra Awakening by Margaret Ann Lembo. Llewellyn Publications, 2011.

The Directory of Essential Oils by Wanda Sellar. The C.W. Daniel Company Limited, 1992.

Energy Healing for Animals by Joan Ranquet. Sounds True, 2015.

Essential Aromatherapy by Susan Worwood. New World Library, Affirmative Books, Ltd., 1995.

The Essential Guide to Crystals, Minerals, and Stones by Margaret Ann Lembo. Llewellyn Publications, 2013.

The Fragrant Mind by Valerie Ann Worwood. New World Library, 1996.

Heal Your Body by Louise Hay. Hay House, 1984.

The Magic of Findhorn by Paul Hawken. Harper & Row, 1975.

Numerology and the Divine Triangle by Faith Javane and Dusty Bunker. Schiffer, 1979.

Bibliography

Ackerman, Diane. *A Natural History of the Senses.* Vintage, 1991.

Alexander, Jane. *The Smudging and Blessings Book: Inspirational Rituals to Cleanse and Heal.* Sterling, 2009.

Andrews, Ted. *Animal-Speak: The Spiritual and Magical Powers of Creatures Great and Small.* Llewellyn Publications, 1993.

———. *Animal-Wise: The Spirit Language and Signs of Nature.* Dragonhawk, 1999.

Aversano, Laura. *The Divine Nature of Plants: Wisdom of the Earth Keepers.* Granite Publishing, 2002.

Bach, Edward, and F. J. Wheeler. *The Bach Flower Remedies Including Heal Thyself; The Twelve Healers; The Bach Flowers Repertory.* Keats Publishing, 1997.

Burnett, Frances Hodgson. *The Secret Garden*. David R. Godine, 1986.

Caddy, Eileen. *The Spirit of Findhorn*. Findhorn Press, 1994.

Cunningham, Scott. *Magical Aromatherapy: The Power of Scent*. Llewellyn Publications, 1989.

Cunningham, Scott, and David Harrington. *The Magical Household: Empower Your Home with Love, Protection, Health, and Happiness*. Llewellyn Publications, 1998.

Davis, Patricia. *Aromatherapy: An A–Z*. The C.W. Daniel Company Limited, 1999.

Gumbel, Dietrich. *Principles of Holistic Therapy with Herbal Essences*. Haug International, 1993.

Hawken, Paul. *The Magic of Findhorn*. Harper & Row, 1975.

Hay, Louise. *Heal Your Body*. Hay House, 1984.

Hickey, Isabel M. *Astrology: A Cosmic Science*. Isabel Hickey, 1970.

Holland, Rob W., Merel Hendriks, and Henk Aarts. "Smells like clean spirit: Nonconscious effects of scent on cognition and behavior." *Psychological Science* 16, 689–693.

Javane, Faith, and Dusty Bunker. *Numerology and the Divine Triangle*. Schiffer, 1979.

Lawless, Julia. *The Encyclopedia of Essential Oils: The Complete Guide to the Use of Aromatic Oils in Aromatherapy, Herbalism, Health, and Well Being*. Conari Press, 2013.

Mahmut, M. K., and R. J. Stevenson. "Olfactory abilities and psychopathy: higher psychopathy scores are associated with poorer odor discrimination and odor identification." *Chemosensory Perception*. doi: 10.1007/s12078-012-9135-7.

Melchizedek, Drunvalo. *Serpent of Light: Beyond 2012—The Movement of the Earth's Kundalini and the Rise of the Female Light, 1949 to 2013.* Weiser Books, 2008.

Milanovich, Dr. Norma, and Dr. Shirley McCune. *The Light Shall Set You Free.* Athena Publishing, 1996.

Miller, Richard Alan, and Iona Miller. *The Magical and Ritual Use of Perfumes.* Destiny Books, 1988.

Nelson Bach. *The Bach Flower Essences® Questionnaire & Guide to Your Own Personal Formula.* Nelson Bach USA Ltd., 1995.

Ouspensky, P. D. *In Search of the Miraculous: Fragments of an Unknown Teaching.* Harcourt Brace Jovanovich, 1949.

Ranquet, Joan. *Energy Healing for Animals.* Sounds True, 2015.

Raven, Hazel. *The Secrets of Angel Healing: Therapies for Mind, Body, and Spirit.* Godsfield Press, 2006.

Rhind, Jennifer Peace. *Fragrance and Wellbeing: Plant Aromatics and Their Influence on the Psyche.* Singing Dragon, 2014.

Sams, Jamie. *The Thirteen Original Clan Mothers: Your Sacred Path to Discovering the Gifts, Talents, and Abilities of the Feminine Through the Ancient Teaching of the Sisterhood.* Harper San Francisco, 1993.

Scheffer, Mechthild. *Bach Flower Therapy Theory and Practice.* Healing Arts Press, 1988.

Schiller, Carol, and David Schiller. *The Aromatherapy Encyclopedia: A Consise Guide to Over 395 Plant Oils.* Basic Health Publications, 2008.

Sellar, Wanda. *The Directory of Essential Oils.* The C.W. Daniel Company Limited, 1992.

Taylor, Terry Lynn. *Messengers of Light: The Angels' Guide to Spiritual Growth.* H. J. Kramer, 1989.

 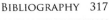

Tisserand, Maggie. *Aromatherapy for Women: A Practical Guide to Essential Oils for Health and Beauty.* Healing Arts Press, 1996.

Tisserand, Robert, and Rodney Young. *Essential Oil Safety,* Second Edition. Churchill Livinstone Elsevier, 2014.

University of Chicago Press. *The Chicago Manual of Style, 16th Edition.* University of Chicago Press, 2010.

Vennells, David. *Bach Flower Remedies for Beginners: A Comprehensive Guide to 38 Essences that Heal.* Llewellyn, 2001.

Virtue, Doreen, and Lynnette Brown. *Angel Numbers: The Angels Explain the Meaning of 111, 444 and Other Numbers in Your Life.* Hay House, 2005.

Webster, Richard. *Spirit & Dream Animals: Decipher Their Messages, Discover Your Totem.* Llewellyn Publications, 2011.

Worwood, Susan. *Essential Aromatherapy: A Pocket Guide to Essential Oils & Aromatherapy.* New World Library, 1995.

Worwood, Valerie Ann. *The Complete Book of Essential Oils and Aromatherapy.* New World Library, 1991.

———. *The Fragrant Mind: Aromatherapy for Personality, Mind, Mood, and Emotion.* New World Library, 1996.

Wright, Machaelle Small. *Perelandra Garden Workbook: A Complete Guide to Gardening with Nature Intelligences.* Perelandra Ltd., 1987.

———. *MAP: The Co-Creative White Brotherhood Medical Assistance Program.* Perelandra Ltd., 1990.

Index

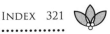

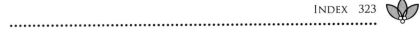

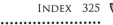

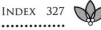

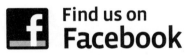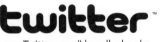

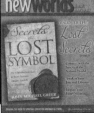

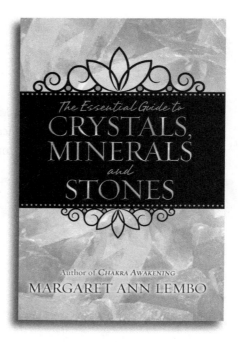

The Essential Guide to
CRYSTALS,
MINERALS
and
STONES

Author of *Chakra Awakening*
MARGARET ANN LEMBO

The Essential Guide to Crystals, Minerals and Stones
MARGARET ANN LEMBO

This ultimate go-to reference features 160 stones you can use to improve your life on all levels—mentally, physically, emotionally, and spiritually. Packed with practical information—from each stone's Mohs scale rating to its divinatory meaning—this unique guide has 190 beautiful full-color photos of specimens commonly found in metaphysical stores. Each page provides concise information: stone name, color, chakra, planet, element, zodiac sign, number, divinatory meaning, and mental, emotional, physical, and spiritual uses. A series of positive affirmations is given for each stone, as well as guidance on how to use gemstones as oracles for personal development and spiritual awakening.

978-0-7387-3252-7, 456 pp., 6 x 9   **$24.99**

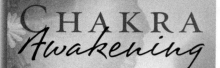

MARGARET ANN LEMBO

CHAKRA
Awakening

TRANSFORM YOUR REALITY USING
CRYSTALS, COLOR, AROMATHERAPY &
THE POWER OF POSITIVE THOUGHT

Chakra Awakening
Transform Your Reality Using Crystals, Color, Aromatherapy & the Power of Positive Thought
MARGARET ANN LEMBO

Bring balance, prosperity, joy, and overall wellness to your life. Use gemstones and crystals to tap into the amazing energy within you—the chakras.

This in-depth and practical guide demonstrates how to activate and balance the seven main chakras—energy centers that influence everything from migraines and fertility to communication and intuition. Perform simple techniques with gems, crystals, and other powerful tools to manifest any goal and create positive change in your physical, emotional, and spiritual well-being.

Chakra Awakening also features color photos and exercises for clearing negative energy, dispelling outdated belief systems, and identifying areas in your life that may be out of balance.

978-0-7387-1485-1, 264 pp., 6 x 9   **$19.95**

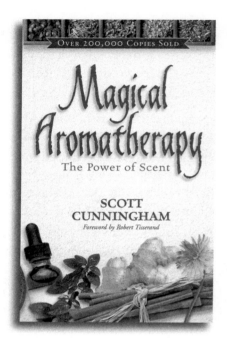

Magical Aromatherapy
The Power of Scent
Scott Cunningham

Scent magic has a rich, colorful history. Today, in the shadow of the next century, there is much we can learn from the simple plants that grace our planet. Most have been used for countless centuries. The energies still vibrate within their aromas.

Scott Cunningham has now combined the current knowledge of the physiological and psychological effects of natural fragrances with the ancient art of magical perfumery. In writing this book, he drew on extensive experimentation and observation, research into 4,000 years of written records, and the wisdom of respected aromatherapy practitioners. *Magical Aromatherapy* contains a wealth of practical tables of aromas of the seasons, days of the week, the planets, and zodiac; use of essential oils with crystals; synthetic and genuine oils and hazardous essential oils. It also contains a handy appendix of aromatherapy organizations and distributors of essential oils and dried plant products.

978-0-87542-129-2, 224 pp., 4³⁄₁₆ x 6⁷⁄₈   **$8.99**

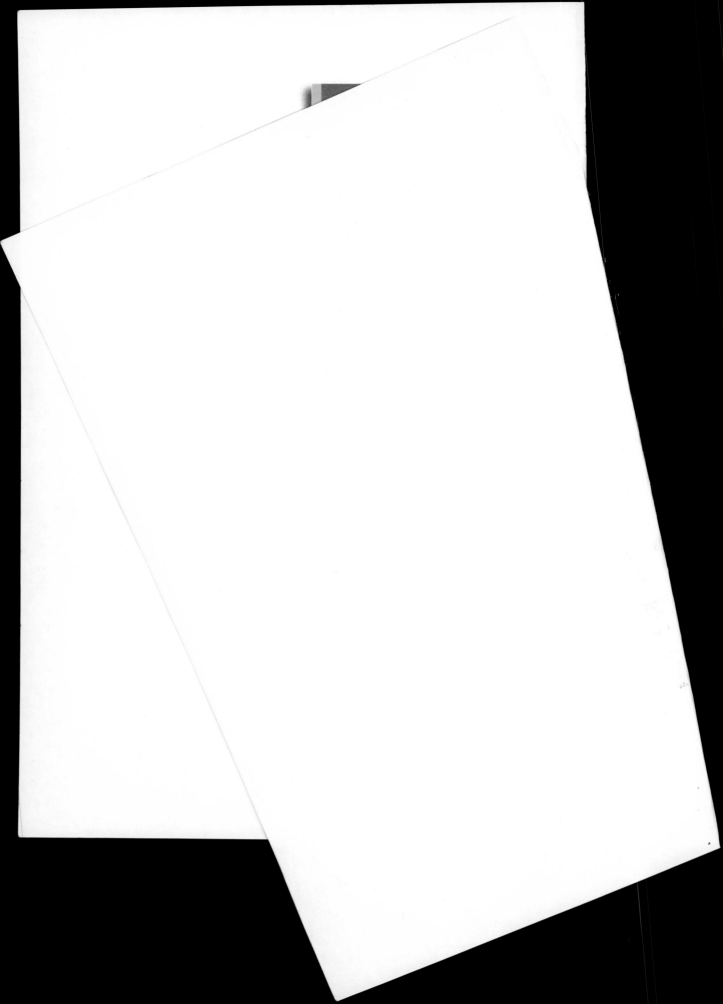

Magical Aromatherapy
The Power of Scent
SCOTT CUNNINGHAM

Scent magic has a rich, colorful history. Today, in the shadow of the next century, there is much we can learn from the simple plants that grace our planet. Most have been used for countless centuries. The energies still vibrate within their aromas.

Scott Cunningham has now combined the current knowledge of the physiological and psychological effects of natural fragrances with the ancient art of magical perfumery. In writing this book, he drew on extensive experimentation and observation, research into 4,000 years of written records, and the wisdom of respected aromatherapy practitioners. *Magical Aromatherapy* contains a wealth of practical tables of aromas of the seasons, days of the week, the planets, and zodiac; use of essential oils with crystals; synthetic and genuine oils and hazardous essential oils. It also contains a handy appendix of aromatherapy organizations and distributors of essential oils and dried plant products.

978-0-87542-129-2, 224 pp., 4³/₁₆ x 6⁷/₈   **$8.99**

To order, call 1-877-NEW-WRLD
Prices subject to change without notice
Order at Llewellyn.com 24 hours a day, 7 days a week

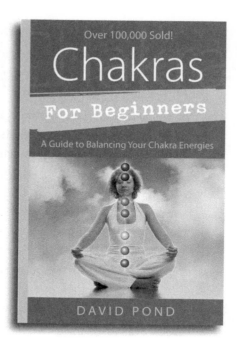

Over 100,000 Sold!

Chakras

For Beginners

A Guide to Balancing Your Chakra Energies

DAVID POND

Chakras For Beginners
A Guide to Balancing Your Chakra Energies
DAVID POND

You may think that difficult situations and emotions you experience are caused by other people or random events. This book will convince you that inner imbalance is not caused by situations in the outer world—instead, your imbalances create the situations that interfere with your sense of well-being and peace.

Chakras For Beginners explains how to align your energy on many levels to achieve balance and health from the inside out. In everyday terms, you will learn the function of the seven body-spirit energy vortexes called chakras. Practical exercises, meditations, and powerful techniques for working with your energy flow will help you overcome imbalances that block your spiritual progress.

- Discover colors and crystals that activate each chakra
- Explore the balanced and unbalanced expressions of each chakra's energies: survival, sexuality, power, love, creativity, intuition, and spirituality
- Practice spiritual exercises, visualizations, and meditations that bring your energies into balance

978-1-56718-537-9, 192 pp., 5³⁄₁₆ x 8   **$13.99**